TEAM-WORK

**This book is to be returned on or before
the last date stamped below.**

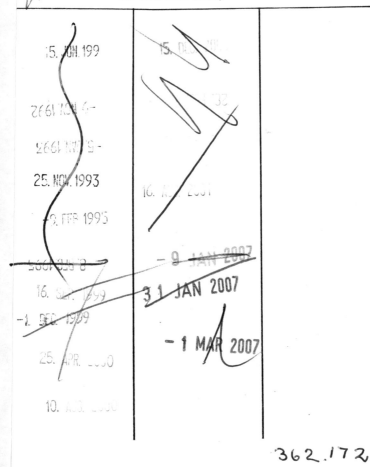

15. JUN. 199

-9 NOV 1992

-5 JAN 1993

25. NOV. 1993

2. FEB 1995

16. SEP. 1999

-1. DEC. 1999

25. APR. 2000

10. AUG. 2000

15. DEC.

16.

- 9 JAN 2007

3 1 JAN 2007

- 1 MAR 2007

362.172

TEAM-WORK
IN
GENERAL PRACTICE

David N. H. Greig MB BChir FRCGP

*General Medical Practitioner and Examiner for
the Royal College of General Practitioners*

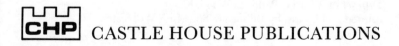 CASTLE HOUSE PUBLICATIONS

To Gillie

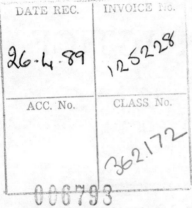
First published in 1988 by
Castle House Publications Ltd
28-30 Church Road
Tunbridge Wells, Kent

British Library Cataloguing in Publication Data

Greig, David
  Team-work in general practice
  1. Family medicine
  I. Title
362.1'72   R729.5G4

ISBN 0-7194-0127-5

Typeset by Vitaset, Paddock Wood, Kent
Printed and bound by Billings & Sons Ltd, Worcester

Contents

Preface

Candidates in the examination for membership of the Royal College of General Practitioners often mention the Primary Health Care Team. One gets the impression that they do not include themselves as members of that team and they conjure up a picture of willing helpers, like a team of enthusiastic huskies ready and willing to pull them out of a tight spot when their own clinical skills, plus a warm heart and hands, have not done the trick.

For many people their only experience of team-work is playing games. There they know what everyone else does and at a pinch could do it themselves. In some cases they may even think they could do it better. Poor team-work then becomes synonymous with not trying hard enough. The situation when delivering health care is somewhat different, firstly because the team is made up of people with widely different skills and attitudes, and secondly because failure to work well as a team means wasted resources and unnecessary suffering for the patients.

Perhaps another reason why team-work is not thought about is because most young health care professionals only experience one primary health care team. If it works well the structure is invisible, it just feels good and people take pride in themselves and their jobs. If it does not work, it hurts. Meetings are dreary and rules seem pointless.

I myself entered General Practice twenty years ago, almost by accident. It has been an interesting time and I have had enormous fun. Much of this pleasure has been because I started at a time when primary health care teams were first being formed. It was, and has been, exciting.

My own training was too narrow in that it was about diseases and not about people. So there was the tremendous excitement and stimulation of learning about the different disciplines and outlook of other people who worked in the community. We also had to learn to work together as a team.

This book is written in the hope that I can pass on some of the fun I have had from working in a team. It is written for general practice vocational trainees who are about to start in their year in the primary health care team, but I hope it will be useful to all the members of the team.

I have sometimes used the pronoun 'he' when writing about doctors and 'she' when writing about other members of the team. This is only because it seems rather longwinded to put he or she every time. There are many more women doctors than there used to be, but men still out-number them. Midwives are always women, as are health visitors, but I am glad to say we are now seeing more male district nurses. We can always hope that one day not only will there be as many men as women, but also that all team members will be equally respected by each other.

David Greig
1988

Acknowledgements

I would like to thank everybody who read through separate sections of the book and made comments on it. Practically every member of my primary health care team read something through and made helpful suggestions. Dr Roddy Hughes and Dr Sue Pocklington both read through the entire manuscript and suggested a number of changes and made many corrections. I adopted most suggestions but any errors in the final draft are my responsibility.

Finally I would particularly like to thank Pam Price who patiently and cheerfully typed and re-typed the whole manuscript and who drew and re-drew most of the diagrams.

David Greig
1988

CHAPTER 1

What is a Primary Health Care Team?

Most people think they know what they mean when they talk about being healthy, but they may have only a vague idea of how to stay healthy or what to do about it if they become ill. The importance placed on health can be gauged by the amount of money that people are prepared to spend on it: in the United Kingdom at the present time the total health care budget is more than £15 000 000 000. The health service employs one person in 50 in the population.

The primary health care team acts as an interface between the general public who provide all the money and the services for which they pay. They can be seen as a filter allowing only those who really need the services access to them. A different view is to think in terms of a general public ignorant of all that a health service can provide for them. It is the job of the primary health care team to make sure that medical care reaches those who need it.

This has worked well in antenatal care, and it is now almost unknown for a woman to have a baby without having been carefully monitored throughout the pregnancy. As a result, the maternal and perinatal mortality rates have fallen to very low levels and will probably fall even lower as special care baby units become more skilled.

Nevertheless, there is still much to be done. Asthmatic children are underdiagnosed and miss much school.[1] Women get pregnant and are not immune to rubella.[2] Many children are not immunised against pertussis. Others are growing up with squints which could have been treated or hearing defects which have made them miss critical learning periods.

Among adults there is undiagnosed hypertension and many women have not had cervical smears taken.[3] Middle-aged people are looking after elderly relatives and, although they would not wish it otherwise, they are often ignorant of what is available to them in the way of money, services and support groups.

Who are the members of the Primary Health Care Team?

This book will deal mainly with those who work from health centres or buildings owned or leased by doctors—that is, people such as general practitioners, health visitors, district nurses, midwives, practice nurses and so on. It is an historical accident that they are based on the general practitioner (GP), and this has some advantages, but it does not mean that the GP has to be the leader of the team. Indeed, who should lead the team depends on the issue. It may be the midwife who institutes combined antenatal clinics in the practice building, or the health visitor who starts up developmental checks or immunisation sessions.

Each member of the team will bring to it their own professional skills, usually with a slightly different approach to that of the others. They will also have different reasons for going into primary health care: some of these will be personal, for instance they may feel that the way of life is easier than in the hospital or in other jobs, or they may feel that they will do more 'good', whatever that may mean. They may also have different scales of priorities, so that for one person it will be just a job, whereas another may approach the task with an almost messianic zeal. All of them are likely to have other interests, homes, families, husbands and so on. These will affect their attitudes to the job.

It is important to recognise that many attitudes are held unconsciously. Working in a team changes attitudes and, unless there is good leadership, there is as much scope for harm as there is for good. A team is a group of people, and people working in groups go through a series of stages in their development that has been well documented. In the first stage they tend to be rather formal with each other as they politely sum one another up. Then they identify differences and struggle for position. Eventually the group either breaks up or agrees on a common task which they settle down to. In due course all groups finish their task and separate. The stages through which groups go are known as forming, storming, norming and mourning. Later on in this book we will be looking at this process in more detail, and identifying where it can go wrong. It is important to realise, however, that if people are going to work together they must be prepared to understand each other, and they must also feel they have some choice about who they are going to work with. The structure of the NHS is such that many people working in it have very little idea how colleagues they see every day spend their time, let alone who pays them and to whom they are responsible. This can mean that they are allocated the wrong tasks by other members of the team.

> One elderly general practitioner spoke to the health visitors only when he wanted somebody to drive out after surgery to give a message or prescription to a patient. He had only a sketchy idea of what their training entailed, and felt it was a breach of confidentiality to let them know if one of his patients became pregnant.

The later chapters in this book will be devoted to describing in outline what the various team members do, what they see as their tasks, and who they think they are responsible to.

Although it rarely happens, it is quite possible for, say, a district nurse or a community psychiatric nurse to be allocated to a GP with little previous consultation. On the face of it this would appear bad. If you have to work in a group you should have some say in who you are going to work with. All the same, it sometimes cannot be avoided as the more the specialist services reach out into the community the more thinly they will have to be spread. Thus the psychiatric nurse who gives very valuable support to patients discharged into the community will often be attached to several practices. One of the problems that primary health care will have to addresss is how to incorporate specialists into the team on a part-time basis. By specialists I do not mean hospital consultants, although there may be room for them as well, but rather people such as audiologists who can and do work very efficiently in the community.

Overview of the book

Delivering primary health care is extremely complicated. Much of what is done seems simple; indeed, it appears to be so simple that it used to be thought that a bit of goodwill and common sense was all that was necessary. The tasks themselves are often straightforward—for instance, sending a letter inviting a patient to come for a cervical smear test or trying to slot a child with earache into a morning surgery. Neither of these needs much training, although both may need a bit of tact. The complexity arises with the multiplicity of tasks and the many different sorts of patients or clients that have to be catered for. It is very difficult to convey to people who have not worked in a primary health care setting just how much is going on and will be continuing to go on day after day and year after year. Somehow the people who provide this care have to be able to pay attention to detail at the same time as retaining a broad view. The structure enabling them to do this must be carefully thought out.

Chapters 1–5 will thus be on underlying structures and tasks. Some generalisation will be inevitable; Chapters 6 and 7 will therefore consider specific tasks with the idea of illustrating the points made in the earlier chapters.

Much team work depends on good communication. Record keeping, being an important part of this, will be considered in Chapter 8. It is an element of performance review which, it is now realised, has a central place in primary health care.

Chapter 11 considers the case conference. This is a well established tool for coping with problems that concern people from different disciplines. In many ways a case conference represents a popular concept of committee work or team work, but they are in fact quite different because their purpose is to allocate responsibility to individuals. Normally committees assume collective responsibility for decisions and have an extended life. A case conference on the other hand may meet only once over one problem and the unwritten rules are therefore different.

The last part of the book will consider members of the team individually to try to give a picture of their jobs as they themselves see them. This section could have been put first as some of the information in it will be assumed in the early chapters. It is intended as a reference section as some of the material will already be familiar to readers of this book.

Disadvantages of basing the primary health care team on the doctor

From the doctor's point of view, and probably from the point of view of the other team members, there are many advantages to the present system, but what does it look like to the patient? Although everybody has a right to a GP, it will not always be the doctor of his or her choice. For example, in some inner cities it has become very difficult to get on to a doctor's list at all. Even in country towns doctors have found that the system of payments has made it progressively less profitable to take on new patients, and once their list size has become big enough they are tempted to demarcate the distances they are prepared to extend their practices and even to refuse to take on the elderly or chronically sick unless forced to do so.

Sometimes a doctor will supply only limited services: for example, some doctors are not willing to do home confinements. There is a letout here because patients can apply to a different GP, specifically for maternity medical services, but the result is that there is fragmentation of both antenatal and postnatal care.

The same sort of situation arises if the doctor, for religious or other reasons, is reluctant to give impartial advice over birth control. The family planning clinics are available but that rather nullifies the concept of a comprehensive service being provided by the same team.

There is also the problem of doctors who, being fiercely independent, find themselves unable to agree strategies of management; whole partnerships may fail to provide adequate services because an individual doctor vetoes them.

What alternatives are available? One that has been tried is putting different independent professionals in the same building, allowing them to practise separately, but hoping they will cooperate and at least give the patients or clients some advantage because of their propinquity. It seems that what then happens is that a proportion of the patients will not use more than one of the professionals on the site and communication is made more difficult.

Teams that go wrong

There is almost no information on what happens to primary health care teams that go wrong. Occasionally a case finds its way to court, or somebody breaks away and sets up on his own. Probably most of the time people just put up with it until, say, a senior partner retires. Even when the team sticks together it may be less effective than it could have been. They may even manage by finding a common outside enemy. Beales, in his book *Sick Health Centres and how to make them better*,[4] describes how two partnerships who moved into a single health centre building managed to get on better among themselves by declaring war on the other partnership. Certainly there are lots of targets about for doctors and nurses to focus their enmity on, such as the bureaucrats at County Hall, hospital doctors, or even the patients. Although there are many reasons why a primary health care team can stop working, the causes can probably be summarised as follows. Members of the team can lose sight of what they are trying to do and, instead of being orientated towards *patient* care, become *team centred*. This may be due to the stress of the job, but also it can be due to confusion because of what seems to be an *impossible* task. They can also simply fail to communicate either formally or informally, or they can lose the will to change.

Table 1.1 compares the characteristics of functional and dysfunctional practices:

Table 1.1 Characteristics of functional and dysfunctional practices

Functional	Dysfunctional
Team takes pride in itself	Unhappy
Aims are defined and agreed	Competitive
Aims are orientated to improving patient care and profits	Scapegoating either internally or externally
Members are emotionally supportive	Rigid rules
Effective	Rigid attitudes
	Ineffective

Changing from a dysfunctional to a functional team depends on identifying that the team is not working and then setting about looking for reasonable aims. This is not easy and is less easy the longer the team has become entrenched in the way it works. Many people will have personal investment in the way things are. It is difficult and galling to admit that, after doing things in a particular way for many years, much energy and frustration could have been saved by doing them differently.

The best way to achieve change is to identify and harness useful aims. In other words, to find out what is being done well in the practice and graft onto it what could be done better.

The inverse care law

The quality of the primary health care team varies widely over the country. It seems that the worst primary health care is in areas of greatest need, for example in inner cities. Such areas are very unattractive to medical staff and the problem is made worse by the fact that the cost of living tends to be much higher. Furthermore, the population changes rapidly, with many temporary residents while there may be many residents from ethnic minorities with poor English, living in squalor. The fact that excellent teams can exist under these circumstances does not detract from the general thesis that the best care is in the areas of least need. The situation has been described as the 'inverse care law'.

This book is directed at all primary health care teams and it is hoped that the principles it discusses will be applicable anywhere; it is, however, appreciated that achieving a high standard is sometimes outside the control of the primary health care team, simply because of lack of resources and the impossible task.

References

1 Speight, A.N.P., Lee, D.A. and Hey, E.N. (1983) Under-diagnosis and undertreatment of Asthma in childhood. *B. Med. J.*, **286**; 1253–6.
2 Smithells, R.W., Sheppard, S., Holzel, H. and Dickson, A. (1985) National Congenital Rubella Surveillance Programme, 1 July 1971–30 June 1984. *B. Med. J.*, **291**; 40.
3 McPherson, A. (1985) Cervical Screening. *J. R. Coll. Gen. Pract.*, **35**; 219–22.
4 Beales, J.G. (1978) *Sick Health Centres and how to make them better*. London, Pitman Medical.

CHAPTER 2

Underlying Structures and Communication

Patient-centred or team-centred?

It may seem superfluous, even impertinent, to point out that the aim of primary health care is to benefit the patient. However, there is ample evidence that in a 'free at the time' health care system there is considerable pressure on the providers, be they doctors, nurses, receptionists, health visitors or whoever, to set up barriers to protect themselves from what they see as unreasonable or even excessive demands. Nobody likes to think that they set up such barriers and it is therefore very easy to deny their existence. When the barriers become too high and the team members feel themselves at risk of being overwhelmed they will begin to lose sight of what they are there for and will start to become team-centred rather than patient-centred in their approach.

I am not arguing that doctors should have an unlimited and open-ended moral contract to serve their patients. What I am saying is that it is up to them to define their relationship with their patients. They have to make up their minds what services they can usefully provide and then make sure they deliver these promptly and effectively. Typical services which they can and should provide are: to be accessible to their patients; to be courteous; and to be sure that they always examine their patients. Patients expect to be examined.[1] A typical service they cannot provide is being a replacement parent or lover. Sometimes there are strong pressures on primary health care workers to do just that. It seems that people who go in for health care professions are often the sort of people who are trying to fulfil unmet needs of their own. In extreme cases it can even develop into what has been called the helping profession syndrome,[2] where the conflict between the need to give support to others and the health care professional's own need for support can finally lead to a breakdown and extreme depression. It is not necessarily a bad thing to go into a profession to meet your own emotional needs; indeed, provided it does not get out of hand there may be a lot to be said for it.

It is somewhere in the grey area between these two opposites of, on the one hand, formal objective provision of base line services, and, on the other, the provision of total emotional support that general practitioners have to decide where to draw the lines. The same arguments apply to the other members of the primary health care team, and once they have decided how far they are prepared to go they are not nearly so much at risk of being overwhelmed.

The members of the team have other needs at a somewhat more superficial but just as realistic a level. They need time and space to do their work. They need breaks when they cannot be watched by clients, but can take coffee and relax and make adverse comments. They usually have homes and hobbies and other preoccupations which have to be respected, including the perfectly respectable desire just to earn a living.

Working in a primary health care team can put further pressure on people because they are seen as possessing power and therefore may become objects of animosity themselves. There are two reasons why they may be seen as powerful figures. The first is that they are seen as gatekeepers to essential, even life saving, services. The second is that they deal with what are regarded as the more intimate aspects of people's lives.

Characteristics of the two approaches

A team-centred approach will therefore embody certain characteristics. The staff will set up barriers between themselves and their clients – for example, they will be anonymous, giving only their surnames. They will make it difficult to arrange appointments either by not being there or by not having appointments available for several days. They will work behind high counters in areas which are inaccessible to the patients and may, for example, store important things such as the patients' notes out of sight. They will wear distinctive uniforms, perhaps white coats, to indicate their separateness and authority.

The patient-centred approach will be the opposite of this, with, for example, staff being readily accessible, encouraging the use of christian names, and allowing patients to read their own notes.

Not making rules

Before leaving the emotional aspect of working in primary health care it is worth pointing out that the whole environment is potentially anxiety provoking. In an average sized practice of say 8000 patients there will be around two deaths per week and the same number of births. Some of these deaths will be unexpected and premature and therefore possibly preventable. Much misery will be seen and from time to time very distressed people will be asked to wait while others are dealt with first. The way in which the team deals with this situation is a measure of how well it functions.

One way is to set up a series of rules. The rules apply to what the team regard as life threatening situations — for example, situations where prompt action can save lives. It might make sense, for example, to ensure that the doctors are informed promptly if a patient has severe chest pain or is an asthmatic unable to control his symptoms. It does not, however, make sense to propound rules for every possible emergency.

Clearly the more rules that are made the less likely it is that they will be remembered and obeyed. Somewhere a compromise has to be found. It is characteristic of organisations where there is much anxiety and little willingness to take responsibility that many rules are made.[3] This can reach extreme proportions: for example, in some hospitals every drug given has to be checked by two qualified nurses and nobody gives the patient clinical information in case it contradicts what they have been told, or will be told, or may be told by the consultant.

There are medical practitioners who, while telling their staff that they must finish their surgeries by a particular time so as to be able to start their rounds, protect themselves by saying they are always willing to see anything urgent. What they fail to do is to define 'urgent' and they thereby delegate responsibility downwards on to their receptionists, who have to make the decision for them. In due course this leads to trouble either between the receptionists and doctors or, worse, between the receptionists and patients, who in their turn will be asked to define urgent.

The only person who is in a position to distinguish medically urgent conditions is the doctor. It is his job and some of his patients will wish to see him simply to learn whether their symptoms are urgent. There is also the question of social urgency. Take the case of a young woman who runs out of contraceptive pills and realises that she is due to start her next pack that evening. Clearly from the social point of view it could be urgent, but all the same she would probably be only too willing to defer to a life threatening medical emergency. Asking her to decide whether she has something urgent is unfair as she needs to know what she is competing against.

Confusing aims and the impossible task

For teams to work they have first to agree on what they are trying to achieve. This is the logical first step which must be taken before going on to decide how they are going to do it.

Negotiating what is important and what the team is trying to do is made particularly difficult because in many cases there are two alternative objectives, both of which may be considered worthwhile but which are mutually incompatible.

The most obvious of these is the conflict between being technological and being human. There are penalties for going to either extreme and much of medicine is to do with striking the correct balance. Technology can often be measured and therefore may get undue emphasis. Being human carries much emotional weight, but it can also pay big dividends by saving resources and time.

Some contrasting demands that have to be decided between are:[4]

1. Technology   *v* Humanity
2. Equity   *v* Excellence
3. Individual   *v* Population
4. Individual performance   *v* Team performance
5. Paternalism   *v* Fraternalism

Technology versus humanity has already been explained.

Equity versus excellence refers to the problem of whether we should concentrate on doing a few things really well, or try to spread our energy over as large an area as possible. It is a daily dilemma and most practices probably feel they get it wrong. Time and energy spent in setting up and running a superb asthma clinic might have been better used checking on the elderly disabled, looking for patients with hypertension, or making sure that patients needing cervical smears are identified. It is possible to go too far the other way and to spread skills so thinly that they become ineffective.

The individual versus the population is another facet of the same thing, except that much emphasis is put on the personal approach in primary health care, and the need to spend time with a particular person. The problem here is that the people who make most use of the primary health care team are often not those most in need. Indeed, the proposal that we send for children to come to screening clincs but bother to examine only those who do not then turn up (by visiting them at home) is not as silly as it sounds. The primary health care team have a responsibility for all the patients on their list, so they have to be careful not to provide too much for the individuals who are most accessible at the expense of those who are not.

Paternalism versus fraternalism. Paternalism is no longer fashionable. All professions are under pressure to share more information with their clients and to share decision making, so medicine, which has always had a reputation for dogmatic assertion, was bound to come under fire. Clearly there is, or has been, a need for more explanation of what and why things are being done to patients. Fraternalism, or the concept of the doctor being on equal terms with the patient and sharing decisions with him, is attractive to those who are healthy and feel in control of their lives. The situation is different when somebody is ill and the decisions to be made are between unpleasant alternatives. People may have to make their own decisions about birth control, but I suspect that few would wish to have to decide whether to have surgery or radiotherapy for their own cancer, especially if they had to learn that neither was statistically likely to be effective. The other risk of fraternalism is that it could be used as an excuse by the doctor to opt out of unpleasant decisions by passing them on to those emotionally unable to cope. Having said that, there are tremendous benefits in clients or primary health care patients participating in decision making about their own health, if only because the majority of them are healthy and decisions they make early in their lives can influence their long term health. For example, not smoking or not becoming obese, can reduce the risk of heart attack.

Marinker has discussed several areas where it is difficult to discern what is the correct objective for a primary care team, and in every team it is likely that the pendulum will swing from one extreme to the other.

Suppressing individual freedom

Working in a team means that sometimes members of the team have to sacrifice their individual freedom in order to make things work.

> Dr Brown had always enjoyed doing obstetrics, largely because of the personal, comfortable relationship he was able to build up with his pregnant women patients over the months before their confinement. He ran no antenatal clinics but liked to fit the patients in during his normal surgery sessions. He regarded the midwife as an encroachment on his freedom and felt that she should do her antenatal care by visiting the patients at home. When his partners set up joint clinics with her he arranged for his cases to be left out and to be seen by himself, sometimes even at his own house. Problems began when he went on his holidays because then his partners insisted on pregnant women being seen with the midwife when she came to the surgery. The midwife would then invite them to the antenatal classes and some of the women were upset to discover what they had been missing. Some also said that they definitely preferred seeing the midwife and meeting other pregnant women. Much time and effort was wasted in resolving these differences.

(Suppressing individuality and agreeing to make protocols work is something which I will come back to later on.)

Another problem occurs when it is difficult to categorise an activity, for example, when a patient has a preventable

Table 2.1   Guaranteed minimum standards

Traditional demand-led general practice

24-hour care for acute illness
Continuity of care
Sorting of undifferentiated problems

Standard management of chronic conditions

Asthma	Hyperuricaemia
Hypertension	Hyperthyroidism

Preventive measures

Antenatal care	Cervical smear screening
Postnatal care	Opportunistic hypertensive screening
Family planning	(Appropriate) geriatric screening
Child health surveillance	

condition which needs effort and time to deal with. Obesity is one such condition, or heavy cigarette smoking.

> Mrs Crimson joined the practice when she moved from London. She brought a letter with her saying that she had had an abnormal cervical smear and the cytologist's report advised a referral for colposcopy. After being seen in the outpatients department she was given a form to fill in at home saying when her monthly periods came on. Despite giving the appearance of being otherwise sensible and intelligent she seemed to find this an impossible task, saying that she was so irregular that it was beyond her ability to write down the day on which she started. The health visitor had to spend much time visiting her and ringing the hospital so that this woman could be admitted on a day when she was not menstruating.

Some GPs do not feel it is part of their job to provide preventive medicine, saying that they are not paid for it except in the case of cervical smears and some immunisations. There may be something in this, as the boundaries between community medicine and general practice have not been clearly drawn. On the other hand, the majority of young GPs and the Royal College of General Practitioners reject this approach, saying that waiting to be paid to do it would imply accepting more external audits and that enforcing minimum standards gives less overall good care than encouraging enthusiasm.

Having said all that, it is probably worth looking at at least one list of minimum standards, which was proposed by a sub-committee of the Newcastle LMC.[5]

Some of these tasks can be allocated to individual team members because they have special skills. Other tasks have been missed off the list but apply to everybody, for example, the job of comforting the sick and unhappy and treating everybody with as much kindness and respect as is possible and appropriate. Many of the tasks could be done by more than one person. Why not have everybody taking blood pressures? Also there are tasks that need the cooperation of more than one person. Teaching mothercraft starts antenatally but is eventually the concern of the health visitor, so the midwife and the health visitor have to liaise.

References

1 Whitehouse, K. (1985) Public Expectations. In: *Health education and general practice*. London, Office of Health Economics. (Discussion document).

2 Malan, D.H. (1979) *Individual psychotherapy and the science of psychodynamics*. London, Butterworth, pp. 131, 139.

3 Menzies, I.E.P. (1977) *Social systems as a defence against anxiety*. London, Tavistock Institute.

4 Marinker, M. (1986) Performance review and professional values. In *Pursuit of quality. J.R. Coll. Gen. Pract.*, 6–14.

5 Brown, A., Jachuck, S.J., Walters, F. and van Zwanenberg, T.D., (1986) The future of general practice in Newcastle-upon-Tyne. *Lancet*, **i**; 370–1.

CHAPTER 3

Communication

Attitudes

When discussing teamwork in Chapter 1, I pointed out that, apart from the professional skills, team members bring with them a number of conscious and subconscious attitudes. Other factors will be important as well, such as liking or disliking other members of the team, loyalty to each member's own peer group, and experience of working in teams.

Let us consider a specific task that the team has identified as useful, leaving aside for a moment the mechanism by which the team will choose the task. Suppose it has been decided that, now that an extra practice nurse has been appointed, it would be useful for most patients with leg ulcers to be treated at the surgery premises. On the face of it this would seem a sensible way of coping with the problem as you would save the district nurse's time. However, they may well not see it that way. Some of the patients they look after would be obvious candidates for changes, such as the old lady who normally does her shopping in town. Others, however, would be less mobile and, although used to visiting, say, their grandchildren by car, would not be totally independent. It is going to be difficult for the district nurse to chivvy such people into coming to the medical centre; the change also carries the implication that the visiting he or she has done in the past was unnecessary. After all, she might argue, dressing leg ulcers is the bread and butter of the district nurse's job, and what will her superiors say if there is a complaint to them? In any case, relieving her of one task may mean that she will be given another more arduous one. She may start asking what advantages there were in getting patients in and may be told that it is easier for the doctor to see the patient with the dressings off. At this point a few subconscious attitudes may be triggered. She may not like the doctor and may think he is a bit lazy. She may feel that the move towards seeing people in medical centres is going too far and that the patients dislike it. There may be some truth in that. Thus the whole project may collapse because the key member who is meant to benefit most does not cooperate and does not send patients in.

It would have been much better if the district nurse had been the prime mover herself; but that is not the point, firstly, because she may be too timid to lead and, secondly, because she is not the only person who is going to benefit from the change. Clearly what was needed was discussion and consensus beforehand. In theory all that is needed is a few meetings, but in practice it does not work like that. It depends on what the team members' previous experience has been of teamwork and of meetings. If they have been used to working in a hierarchical structure meetings may be equivalent to briefings, in which they are given instructions but no say in the matter. They may even have gone into district nursing in order to get away from such meetings.

Communication

Formal and informal meetings and communication in general

Are meetings and those who go to them time wasting, boring and ineffective? They easily can be and they often are.

It is often not realised that people have to learn about meetings and about how to use them. Time is such a precious commodity that it is a tragedy to waste it. If it cannot be used effectively then surely it should be spent in enjoyment and not in boring, boring meetings? The answer is that those who go to meetings should learn how to make them work, and there is much to learn.

Informal meetings

Much can be done in a medical centre by structuring timetables and architecture to foster informal meetings. The traditional work pattern for a GP used to be to start morning surgery at 9.00 am, work through a list of patients, take a cup of coffee

Figure 3.1 Leader's programme

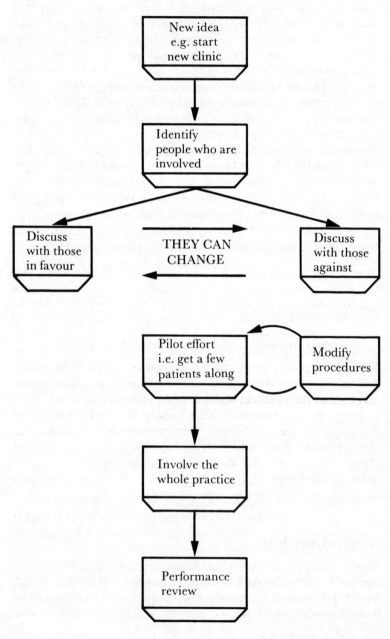

while receiving messages or making telephone calls, and then leave to do visits by car. Even when there are only a couple of doctors working in a building this system might have meant that, because they had different lengths of surgery, the two doctors could go several weeks without ever meeting each other. Team members have only to commit themselves to coffee at a set time, say 10.30 each morning, and they will be able to exchange worries, information and problems on a daily basis so that nothing can reach crisis point without due warning. The alternative to sitting down in a coffee room can easily degenerate into an erratic system of people trying to catch each other when they are most preoccupied with other things. It can easily degenerate into a situation where health visitors lie in wait for the doctors at the end of their surgeries, waiting to pounce out for hurried discussions about patients.

Passing on information without using meetings

Sometimes meetings are used to pass on information that can be better conveyed by notices and charts. For example, it was a regular complaint of one district nurse that nobody told her if a patient had died in the night or been suddenly admitted to hospital. This meant that she would then be put in an embarrassing position if she did a routine housecall the following day to give treatment. A book provided for messages tended to be used for instructions rather than information. Eventually the problem was solved by putting up a blackboard in the corridor leading to the coffee room. Deaths, admissions to hospital, who was on leave and much other information could then be written on it in bold letters.

Formal meetings

People have meetings for all sorts of reasons, so what are meetings good for? Do they, for example, foster team spirit? If they do it may be worth while having meetings just in order to do that. Certainly when people are put into unstructured groups there is a tendency for them to become more friendly. It seems that it is a natural tendency among human beings, which can reach bizarre proportions as happens when people who have been held hostage get so friendly with their captor that

Table 3.1 Meetings held in a typical practice

Meeting	Present	Discussion
Weekly management	2 Partners Practice manager Practice nurse Senior receptionist	Administration Troubleshooting
Monthly partners' meeting	All partners Practice manager (who does not come when they are clinical meetings)	Policy decisions and finance
Quarterly primary health care team	All partners Practice manager Practice nurse Health visitors Midwife Community psychiatric nurse	Policy decisions and communication

they afterwards feel the need to visit him in prison. This does not, however, always happen in real life and it seems that there is also a tendency for people to try to check this progress towards intimacy unless they feel that in due course the group is going to break and they can get away. Small groups do have a use in medical practice, but it is not in the formal running of the medical centre.

Useful meetings

The principal uses of meetings are:

- To share information that cannot be shared in other ways.
- To achieve democratic decisions and agree strategy.
- To ask for specialist advice.
- To give instructions.
- Buzz groups.

Most formal meetings have all these functions and it is the confusion about which particular function they are fulfilling at a particular moment that can make them ineffective. It is the job of the chairman to know what the purpose of the meeting is at any point and to make sure that the people at the meeting know what they are doing.

Sharing information that cannot be shared in other ways

Talking to more than one person at a time is an ineffective way of giving out information. Most people listen until they reach a place where they do not agree with what is being said, and then wait for an opportunity to chip in with what they want to say. While they wait they do not listen. This is why it is useful for reports and discussion papers to be circulated before meetings. Members of the committee can then read them and make sure they understand what is going on before arriving at the meeting. If somebody asks for factual information at a meeting that he could have got beforehand for himself he will be wasting the time of everybody there who already has the information.

Sometimes information is confidential. It is not therefore appropriate to write it down. For example, there may be personal problems among the staff that need to be talked through. Sometimes information is very unwieldy and it may be easier to exchange it face to face. For example, agreeing on an 'on call' rota is easiest when everybody who is involved is there to negotiate.

Achieving democratic decisions and agreeing strategy

Where people do not have the same voting power a meeting can evolve into a situation where some members are giving orders to others. It is not always black and white because, although, say, a general practitioner and his receptionist may both be at the meeting, no matter how much authority the GP has he cannot make his receptionist do what is unworkable. Thus the receptionist's special skills have some power and influence in what happens as only she knows what would or would not be workable.

By the time the issue gets to a formal meeting the problems should have been thought through. The meeting itself then becomes a straightforward matter of rubber stamping something that has already been decided. This has its merits, firstly, because it formalises the situation that may have been fluid and, secondly, because if everyone who is involved in a change is present, then the decision is given collective responsibility. That is to say, it has been agreed and, however badly it turns out later, nobody can blame somebody else.

The casual observer at a meeting might think that what occurs is that a new idea is presented, it is discussed and a rational decision is made. In fact when it involves a radical change it is only a very experienced and mature group who are able to do this effectively. Generally speaking, those in favour of the new idea will remain silent whereas those who are affected most and who may feel most vulnerable do much of the talking. This can give the impression that everybody is against a change. The chairman's job is to identify the mood of the meeting. He or she has to isolate the most important issues and draw them to the attention of the meeting. If necessary he may have to take a vote. He has to be wary of passing a motion where there is a narrow majority because there may be so many people who do not agree that it will make the project unworkable even though the decision was a democratic one on paper. A good chairman will sense when this is going to happen and try to defer taking a vote until another meeting, by which time the people will have had more time to sort out their position. This is usually possible in a primary health care team because administrative decisions rarely have to be made against a deadline.

CHAPTER 4

Other Sorts of Meetings

Meeting the specialists from outside and taking advice

When a piece of new equipment is installed or the team needs to think about outside resources it is often easier to call a meeting so that everyone can get the information at the same time. There is only a very limited amount of information that can be transmitted in this way, partly because of the difficulty of getting everyone together. There is also the problem that only a certain amount of information can be transmitted in a given time; where a lot of information is going to be given a handout beforehand may be necessary. The meeting with the expert can be used as a questioning and answering session. A good time to have such meetings is at 8.30 in the morning with a half hour time limit. If they are held later in the day there is a tendency for the person bringing information to drift on over the time limit set.

Buzz groups and brainstorming

Buzz groups are a special form of meeting. They are sometimes used in industry to generate new ideas. They probably have little application in primary health care if used in their most basic form. The technique is that everybody throws in ideas and one person only is a scribe who notes them down. The only rule is that, although people may amend or add to what others say, they may not criticise. In this way it is possible to generate fresh ideas and then at the end of the meeting to sort out those that can be used. A buzz group is not a foolproof method for solving problems but it can produce surprising and interesting new ideas, often because something thrown in frivolously actually fits the problem or at least triggers a solution.

It is likely that the most valuable use of buzz groups for

people working in primary health teams is that, if they have experience of them, they will learn to listen for and to new ideas less critically. That is not to say that there is no place for criticism, but rather that it should be constructive. Working in buzz groups helps people to add on to new ideas which may be useful rather than wasting time looking for flaws in an idea that has already been suggested.

Making changes in management

It is a characteristic of effective management that there is continuous change. This sometimes surprises people who seem to expect a reorganisation to be a once and for all activity which will solve all problems. That cannot be so as the external world is continuously changing. There are changes in the structure of the population being looked after, there are changes in the management of disease as new scientific discoveries are made, and there are changes in outlook by professionals in the primary health care team as new insights are gained.

Over the next few years it seems likely that, as the number of elderly patients continues to increase, the emphasis of primary care will move towards planned prevention and towards the management of chronic disease. It also seems likely that computerisation of practices and family practitioner committees will mean more team as against patient initiated activities. There will also be a move towards consumerism. This has already affected other professionals such as solicitors and will undoubtedly begin to affect general practitioners and all primary health care professionals.

Some organisational changes just happen, but most of them need something more to make them work. They need planning and leadership. Anyone in the primary health care team can be the leader, but it is usually expected to be one of the general practitioners. There is now a move afoot for general practitioners and their practice managers to go to management courses.

Leadership is an exercise in determination, tact and planning. It is not enough to have a good idea. Most good ideas are automatically rejected by the people involved because most people do not like change. The leader therefore has to go through a series of stages. Firstly, he or she has to think through what he wishes to achieve and why. He has to identify who will be involved and make some sort of assessment as to whether they will be for or against the changes. He then has to sound out the people involved to find out what their actual position is and talk it through with them. The next phase is to present the concept to the whole group, preferably in a fairly low key way and perhaps try it out on a small scale. If it works it can then be offered to everybody. Several things will happen. People will change from being for the idea to being against it. They will also change from being against it to being for it. The original idea may get modified. There will be antagonism by some people, and unless the leader continues to monitor progress, the new initiative will be lost. As Sally Fountain describes the problem:

> The art of coordinating all these contributions to a common end is intrinsic to good management. It is about companionship, teamwork and leadership. Teamwork is the means whereby people work with concentrated effort to reach a common goal. To achieve full cooperation and to be able to monitor and control disparate activities and people to a single end point requires a leader who exudes self-confidence and optimism, while being highly considerate of human relations. He has to be powerful and popular at the same time. He has to be strong when necessary and yet permissive when the occasion demands.[1]

In later chapters I will be looking at some successful initiatives, especially in the management of chronic disease. All new ideas do not always work. In one practice I know of they changed to A4 records, but because the system was not properly monitored the advantages were soon dissipated and the larger record folders became as disorganised as the previous Lloyd George ones, but the mess was now bigger and so the records became more difficult to use than they had been before the change.

In another practice a partner tried to introduce a system of individual as against shared lists but met with such antagonism that the whole thing had to be dropped until the senior partner had a myocardial infarction and had to retire. The partner who had wanted to change then got his way, but it was at the cost of feeling accused of causing his senior's heart attack.

Reference

1 Fountain, S. (1986) Management in practice. In: *Medical Annual*. Bristol, Wrights, p. 258.

CHAPTER 5

Minutes, Reports, Profits, Size

Minutes of meetings and practice reports

Somebody, somewhere, described a committee as a place for keeping minutes but wasting hours. Somebody else described a practice report as an ideal way of generating orphan data. By orphan data he meant that mass of statistics that are collected but never used or never read. Both of these statements have some truth in them, but all the same there are very good reasons indeed for keeping minutes of meetings in a primary health care team and others that are as good for having a practice report. Despite these, many otherwise sophisticated practices have neither.

The sorts of change that occur in a professional team tend to be rather amorphous developments. This is desirable because it lets everybody get used to a new idea. On the other hand, when there are competing policies it is essential that they should sometimes be formalised and discussed. This can happen only in a meeting and the conclusion of the meeting must then be minuted. At subsequent meetings the decision can then be read out, confirming it or giving people another chance to amend it. This sounds like a statement of the obvious, but it is impossible to overestimate the value of good minutes. They are like stepping stones in the process of development of the team and protect everyone from misunderstandings. The person who writes the minutes is even more powerful than the chairman, whose only prerogative is to choose the agenda and have a casting vote.

A practice report

Whereas minutes are well tried and accepted, practice reports are a relatively new concept.[1] A practice report is a different sort of document and includes a variety of statements, which,

Figure 5.1 What the practice report should illustrate

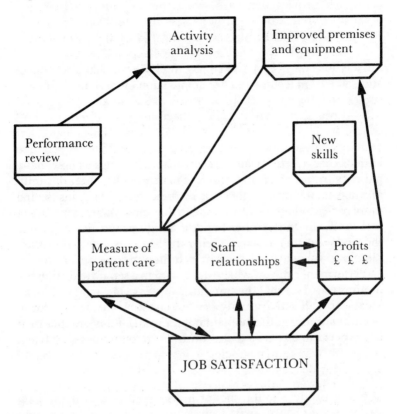

by implication, are important for practice policy; in this way it gives guidelines on what is being, or has been, achieved.

Contents of the practice report

The minutes and the practice report can be seen as complementary to each other. The practice report is the instrument of leadership; the minutes of the regular meetings confirm what is and has been achieved.

In most businesses the success of the operation can be measured by the profits. If it is making money it must be a success; the only question then remaining will be whether the business will continue to make money. In a primary health care

team there is a need to make profits but there is also a need to provide and improve patient care beyond the minimum that is needed
to satisfy the terms and conditions of service. No business can survive, however, unless the people running it feel that it is worthwhile
—in other words, that they get job satisfaction. Some of this job
satisfaction comes from working with people you like and respect
and some from feeling you are doing a good job. Some of it even
comes from the pay packet, but less than is generally assumed.

The practice report should reflect these requirements and
should try to do so in a way that makes sense. This means that
activity analyses must be interpreted to show that they relate to
patient care. (Activity analysis means such things as how many
patients are seen, how many house calls are made, what are immunisation scores, or how good the records are.) Clearly just seeing
more patients does not always mean that more patients are better
looked after. On the other hand, if a high proportion have had
their cervical smear taken, their rubella status assessed or their
blood pressure checked, they are definitely getting better care.

Performance review will be dealt with in a separate section but
its aims are to see that the standards set are being achieved. In an
ideal world all activity analysis would be subjected to a performance review, but at the moment it is unusual for any practice to be
doing performance review on more than one or two aspects of care.

Profits

What attitude should the primary health care team have
towards the profits, apart from sympathy and concern for the
partners if they fall? The rest of them are, after all, paid on an
independent scale. The turnover and the profits are probably
the legitimate concern of everybody. Rightly or wrongly, if they
fall the partners will feel undervalued, even though the reasons
why they fall may be outside their control and more to do with
government policy. They are therefore likely to respond to even
a relatively small loss of income by cutting back on expenses,
which include maintenance of the premises, new equipment
and even staff pensions or bonuses. Whether it is right that
general practitioners should be paid the way they are, and it is
an issue which I will address from time to time in this book,
there is no question that increased profits are more likely to
improve everybody's job satisfaction.

What is the best size for a primary health care team?

Everything that has been said so far could apply to a practice of almost any number of partners, but this does not mean that all points apply with equal force to all the different sorts of practices that exist. Although there is much to be said for a single-handed doctor writing an annual practice report, there is considerably more need for one in a practice with half-a-dozen doctors.

The single-handed doctor has many advantages. His team is smaller, and therefore policy changes can be made more easily. Communication is easier because fewer people have to be accommodated. There is likely to be a smaller list of patients to look after so trouble spots are known to the whole team. On the other hand, the doctor has problems getting time off, he has problems if he is sick, and he is dependent on getting locums if he wants to go on holiday. He also lacks the stimulus of a peer who can keep him up to date and provide new ideas.

At the other extreme there are practices of more than half-a-dozen doctors where, unless there is an extremely powerful leader, it is difficult for any change to be made and they just drift according to the whims of chance and government pressure. In between are the majority with two or three doctors, but here again there can be problems because there are clashes of personality in small practices which cause breakdowns that would be cushioned if there were more people in the partnership. In my view it is very rare for doctors in small partnerships to get on well over many years. It is a bit like a marriage — if there are no quarrels it is likely that one partner is dominant and the other(s) always give(s) way. Disagreements in themselves are no bad thing, it is how they are resolved and whether they can be resolved that matters. Three people are less likely to reach a deadlock than two because the third can have a casting vote. If there are three partners the total number of people working in the building will be manageable at about a dozen. Once you get over five the numbers are too big for easy contact and communication.

Reference

1 Pereira-Gray, D. (1985) Practice annual reports. In: *Medical Annual*. Bristol, Wrights, p. 282.

CHAPTER 6

What the Team Does – I

The tasks of the team

In Chapter 2 the problem of deciding on appropriate tasks for the team was introduced. This chapter will discuss the topic in more detail.

The tasks of the team can be divided into:

- acute intervention in disease,
- the long term management of disease,
- screening, and
- prevention of illness.

Time and energy spent on one activity cannot be used on another.

There is, or was, a widely held belief that medical carers have no control over demand for their services and the failure of the NHS is thus blamed on limited resources trying to cope with unlimited demand. We will be looking at this concept to see how true it is. If it is wrong it is the responsibility of the health service worker to look carefully at how he or she spends his or her time. It is also important to look at ways of being more effective.

Patient demand and acute intervention

The acceptance of problems as suitable for medical care depends on many signals given by the doctor and receptionists. In the past 10 years there has been a change in the way the general public respond to influenza, the tendency now being not to call the doctor until the illness has had two or three days' run.

It is easy to think of reasons for this change: there have been changes in certification rules, advertisements on television and a loss of faith in antibiotics. When an epidemic starts it is usually announced on television coupled with advice on what home remedies to use and when to call the doctor. So how much effect does an individual practitioner's behaviour have on the way his services are used?

A study on this topic was done by Howie & Hutchinson in a Scottish practice,[1] where they compared the consultation rate for small children between three partners in the same practice, one of whom believed in giving antibiotics to all children with upper respiratory tract infections whereas his partners used this treatment rarely. Presumably the first partner felt that antibiotics would shorten the disease and patients would be less likely to come back. In fact more of his patients came back, usually because the medicine had not worked within 24 hours. Whatever else had happened he had created a different set of *expectations* for his patients to those created by his partners.

It is a common observation that doctors who diagnose tonsillitis frequently see a lot of patients with sore throats and give them penicillin. Yet there is evidence that penicillin has little effect on the length of symptoms in the acute phase,[2] and even less on the long term symptoms. It seems that the expectations raised are an important factor and that the expectations are sometimes created by doctors.

A further point is that the doctors' own ideas of what they should treat will change. A few years ago it was widely accepted that counselling and marriage guidance were part of the general practitioner's job, until it was pointed out that overenthusiastic probing into the psyche of unwilling patients amounted to 'mind rape'.[3] The fashion died out.

Sometimes a *deliberate policy* will change the pattern of acute intervention. If the practice nurse agrees to see patients with cuts, bruises and scrapes the receptionists will start directing patients towards her. Equally, however, the pattern of management of acute episodes of illness can be changed just by *serendipity*. The health visitor tends to be the member of the team who does most weighing of babies. When small children have diarrhoea and vomiting they are therefore often seen by the health visitor who, after weighing them, would help monitor their treatment. Within a short time the health visitor herself will be managing all cases of infant diarrhoea and vomiting. In a way this is a natural bridge from feeding problems.

It is worth acknowledging this underlying trend if only to see whether it is appropriate. If there is an increase in demand for health check-ups it is worth deciding what sort of check-ups are of value and how they should be done.

Accessibility and acute intervention

There is some evidence that primary health care teams are reaching those who need them most. There is also evidence that social class V patients use the primary health care team more than people of other social classes. This again is encouraging as both morbidity and mortality are highest in social class V. Unfortunately, however, the use of the primary health care team by the lower classes is still not matched by the amount of extra illness they have.[4]

One complaint made by many patients is that they find it difficult to get an appointment to see their doctor. Even when they get an appointment they are kept waiting. Providing a poor service during the day means that patients defer seeing the doctor or nurse and call them out in a panic after hours. One measure of bad day time care and inaccessibility by the doctor is the number of late evening calls the practice gets.

The best time to see and deal with medical problems is during the period between 9.00 am. and 5.00 pm. People can be seen in daylight, laboratories are open to accept specimens, and X-ray departments are open to make appointments or give results of investigations over the telephone. Yet many doctors still start their evening surgeries at 5.00 pm, sometimes after spending much of the afternoon doing nothing.

Although the advantages of not working late are clear for the doctor and his receptionists, the usual counter when such a system is proposed is that many patients cannot come to see their doctor because they themselves are at work. The main

Table 6.1   Influences on pattern of acute intervention

1.   Public announcements – TV etc.
2.   Doctors and the expectations they raise
3.   Changes in availability of other team members
4.   Availability and accessibility
5.   Emphasis

users of the health service are, however, the elderly (and retired) and young mothers with children. A few employers refuse to give time off work to see the doctor, so some provision has to be made for non-urgent consultations by working people. The sensible method is for the duty partner for that day to run a later surgery. Pregnant women have a legal right to miss work to go to antenatal clinics.

It is the stated policy of the Royal College of General Practioners that all patients should always be able to see their own doctor. Under normal circumstances it should be possible to provide appointments that enable non-urgent patients to see the doctor of their choice within the day, and usually at the next surgery.[5] An essential component of running such a service is that the doctors use a system of personal lists.

Personal lists

In some practices the patients may be registered with one doctor but free to see any doctor who is available and willing to see them. This can happen in a practice when the number of patients being looked after gets too large for the existing partners and a new doctor is taken on. While he is building up his own practice it is only sensible that he should help out the others by seeing some of their patients. Problems arise because what happens is that no individual takes responsibility for the care of a particular patient and there tends to be a loss of continuity.

The 'collusion of anonymity' is the name given to the situation that arises when a patient, or a family of patients, gets lost between partners.[6] Such patients usually come from a poorer part of the practice and are generally unattractive, either because they are dirty and stupid or because they are difficult. They shift from one doctor to another to another, none of whom particularly likes them and all of whom assume that another partner has taken responsibility. As the patient often has the most severe problems in the practice they are therefore doubly disadvantaged.

Many doctors regard continuity of care as one of the strengths of general practice. It is possible to devise a scale which measures how often patients registered with one doctor actually see another. Where a practice has a personal list system they should see another doctor only on those rare occasions when their own doctor is away, or when the problem is of such a personal nature that they would like to see, say, somebody of their own sex. One study showed that where there was a combined list system the chances of seeing the same doctor on two successive occasions was only 50%.[7]

The issue is not black and white. There are patients who have no objection to seeing any doctor and there are practices whose members find it very difficult to make sense of an appointment system and who eventually abandon it on the grounds that it is better to see patients who do not mind waiting without any appointment than have everybody wait for several days.

So far the discussion has referred to doctors, but continuity of care is as important for other members of the team. If there is more than one health visitor the simplest system is probably to divide the practice into geographical areas, adjusted according to workload. Problems arise when too many health visitors work from the same building and it becomes difficult for other people in the team to remember which area is being covered by which health visitor.

Although health visitors may see some patients by appointment—for example, when doing developmental assessments— they usually also operate clinic days where there is open access. This has the advantage that they can see clients together and when one is away they at least have some information about problems normally in the other's patch.

Emphasis

It may be that the biggest influence of all in changing patterns of use of the team is the amount of emphasis that doctors attach to different symptoms. Byrne and Long showed that the most constant factor in a consultation was the doctor.[8] It seems likely that each doctor accepts only a limited range of problems as suitable for him to deal with, rejecting the rest. Patients tend to have contact with only a few doctors in their lives and their expectations of doctors will therefore be based on this fairly limited experience.

Although it is difficult to measure this influence, modifying help-seeking behaviour is definitely part of the doctor's role. Stott & Davis pointed out that it is an essential component of every consultation.[9]

References

1 Howie, J.G.R. and Hutchinson, K.R. (1978) Antibiotics and respiratory illness in general practice: prescribing policy and work load. *Br. Med. J.*, **ii**; 1342.

2 Whitfield, M.J. and Hughes, A.O. (1981) Penicillin in sore throat. *Practitioner*, **225**; 234–9.

3 Zigmond, D. (1978) When balinting is mind rape. *Update*, **16**; 1123–6.

4 Crombie, D.L. (1984) Social class and health status. Equality or difference. McConaghey Memorial Lecture, 1984. *R. Coll. Gen. Pract.*, Occasional Paper 25.

5 Greig, D.N.H. (1984) Making an appointments system work. *Br. Med. J.*, **288**; 1423–5.

6 Balint, M. (1952) *The doctor, his patient and the illness*. London, Pitman Medical, 2nd Ed. 1974, 69–80.

7 Fishbacker, C.M. and Robertson, R.A. (1986) Patients' difficulties in obtaining appointments—a general practice audit. *J. R. Coll. Gen. Pract.*, **36**; 282–4.

8 Byrne, P.S., and Long, B.E.L. (1976) *Doctors talking to patients*. London, H.M.S.O.

9 Stott, N.C.H., and Davis, C.H. (1979) The exceptional potential in each primary care consultation. *J. R. Coll. Gen. Pract.*, **29**; 201–5.

CHAPTER 7

What the Team Does – II

Prevention

Prevention of disease is clearly the responsibility of the primary health care team, but it is interesting to see how ideas have changed over the last decade. It used to be thought that there was much undiagnosed but treatable disease in the community which, if caught early by doing a formal screening programme, could be treated to prevent problems later. The issue boils down to a question of costs and benefits. The cost of identifying very few unknown cases of an illness can make it hardly worth while screening most of the population, although a case could perhaps be made for the elderly. On the other hand it has been pointed out that most patients are seen by GPs several times in a year and the health workers who see them are in a unique position to do such things as measure blood pressure.

When thinking about the possibility of prevention the amount of effort involved has to be weighed against the benefit over a relevant time span. Sometimes a limited sum of money is available on a one off basis. When it is used up there is little incentive to go on, and people lose interest.

The primary health care team can expect a long life. Some of the benefits of prevention could actually accrue to the team members—for example, persuading a mother to breast-feed instead of bottle-feed could cut down on the demands that that mother makes on the service in the first few months of her baby's life. Identifying high blood pressure may save the GP work later on because he will have fewer stroke patients to care for. At the absolute extreme, benefit may extend into the next generation—for example, there is evidence that depression in young women is directly related to their social circumstances,[1] and it seems likely that depression could affect their mothering skills or even lead to marital breakdown, all consequences for the next generation. The primary health care team can certainly help the children of divorce by talking to the parents about not using their children as pawns in the marital warfare, and explaining to them that children need to know that the divorce is not their fault.

Diet is another important area. Obesity causes preventable death from cardiovascular disease. It seems, however, that the amount of influence that outsiders such as primary health team workers exert is limited because a large component of obesity is hereditary[2] and motivation by the sufferer is extremely important; indeed, long term follow up of the obese is extremely disappointing. It is now believed that diet is a more important cause for concern than is cigarette smoking,[3] but unfortunately the rapid changes in stance taken by the medical professions as new research has changed ideas has made them lose some

Table 7.1

Effort	*Objective*	*Benefit*
About 5 minutes per patient by receptionist, least qualified lowest salary member of team	Rubella immunity in all women on the pill	Could save severe and lifelong disability
Questionnaires or high level of suspicion by member of team with highest salary and longest training	Identify problem drinker	Good results with early social drinker ineffective with many drinkers
Continuous low grade effort by health visitor	Modification of mothering behaviour	Benefits could extend into next generation
Continuous low grade effort by health visitor and others	Stopping an adolescent smoking	May prevent lifelong addiction and add 5% to life expectation
High index of suspicion needed. Biochemical tests	Identifying patients hypercholesterol-aemia	Reduction in a few deaths in young people

credibility with the general public. The likely benefits of any preventive activity can be listed and compared with the effort needed to achieve them, as in Table 7.1.

It can be seen that there is no clear cut hierarchy of priorities, but, broadly, a team would be sensible to make sure they have a good strategy for identifying women at risk for rubella in pregnancy before they start making up protocols for finding early alcoholics.

The potential of every consultation

Stott and Davis have pointed out that every consultation has the potential for opportunistic health promotion.[4] This need not be very elaborate or time consuming, but can be very effective. It is more valuable, however, if followed up by offers of support; for example, if people decide to stop smoking or lose weight. Compare two health workers who go into work one morning. A practice nurse who persuades a young patient it is worth stopping smoking is probably doing more good than a thoracic surgeon doing a coronary bypass graft. Clearly the nurse has given the patient a more useful and healthy life than has the surgeon. Both patients may be suffering from the same disease, addiction to cigarettes.

Long term management

As diabetes, hypertension and asthma continue for many years and therefore need special strategies for their management, both doctor and patient have to come to terms with the illness. Once a patient has settled into a pattern of coping with such an illness it is very difficult to change it. At the moment we do not know much about preventing these diseases so we have to identify those patients who have them and try to give them the best possible care. There are two separate stages in this. All cases must first be diagnosed and, second, be put on a register so their management can be audited.

Consider the patients in the practice with diabetes. Some will be undiagnosed and they may or may not have symptoms. Others will know they have diabetes but be determined to control themselves, for instance by diet. Neither of these two groups will come to much harm, although they may suffer some discomfort. There will then be a further group who will be known to have the disease but, through ignorance, indolence, obstinacy or fear, do not look after themselves properly; such people will include the young insulin dependent diabetic who continuously defaults on appointments with the ophthalmic surgeon, and the elderly woman who finds it almost impossible to lose weight. The next group will be the 'good' patients. They will come to the doctor or the practice nurse in a clinic and will take advice. These patients will benefit most of all from special protocols set up by the practice but are less at risk than the other groups. Then there is a further group who take their disease extremely seriously. These people insist on going to the hospital diabetic clinic. They are methodical and careful. We believe that the outlook for these is better than for other patients and there is evidence to support this belief,[5, 6] but even these patients will suffer complications.

Each of these different categories of patients poses different problems for the primary health care team in the allocation of resources. Take those patients who are undiagnosed but uncomfortable. Should we screen the practice to try to identify them? How much energy should we use to do this?

The next category is more difficult still. If patients are ignorant about their disease whose fault is it? They certainly make us feel guilty and in some cases perhaps rightly so. On the other hand, we can take this too far. Part of our job must surely be to give patients autonomy and not to create dependence.

We then get to the 'good' patients, the ones who come to the clinics. Here we have another duty, which is to make sure that we waste neither their time nor ours. We have to think through what we are going to do in a clinic before we set it up. When thinking about whether to start a diabetic clinic in our practice we thought very carefully about the form the flow sheet should take and asked ourselves what would be the most useful things to put on it. We decided that the single most useful thing we could do would be to stop diabetics smoking and that taking a single random blood sugar sample was a waste of time. It was only worth while taking blood sugar concentrations through the day with BM stix or on blotting paper strips. We therefore designed our chart with these items put in prominent positions. We did not include routine testing of vibration sense as we felt this was of little value.

The advantages for the team in having a clinic are that the

staff can prepare themselves so that they are mentally geared up for the patients, they can have special equipment out and ready, and they can bring in experts, such as the dietician, especially for that clinic. They also feel that they are getting to grips with things. The disadvantage is that the clinics may be more time consuming than just seeing the patients at ordinary surgery attendances.

The advantages for the patient are more nebulous. He or she probably gets more intensive and therefore better care, but against this he or she has to come at a particular and possibly inconvenient time. He may see the nurse or doctor he does not particularly want to see. He may dislike going to clinics where he knows that everybody knows that he is a diabetic (admittedly not as bad as attending a family planning clinic where everybody knows why you are there) and he may dislike not being able to raise other problems at the same time as he comes to the clinic. Sometimes it is very difficult for women with small children to get to the surgery and therefore it is very irksome to have to make two journeys, for example to come to an antenatal clinic and then again, perhaps later in the day, to a surgery with an ailing child.

Management of special groups of patients

Chronic Illness

There are certain underlying principles in the management of chronic diseases:

1. *Set out the objectives*
What exactly do you hope to achieve when managing a chronic illness? Clearly the aim should be that the patient or client should have as normal and as long a life as possible. So much is obvious and generally accepted, but when it comes to writing down the practical details it is less easy. The situation is rarely clear cut and either the doctor or the patient may have to make choices between some inconvenience or discomfort and added risks. One patient may prefer to feel a little sleepy on his beta-blockers than risk a stroke or possible side-effects if he changes to another drug for his hypertension. Another may find the side-effects of any treatment intolerable.

The team has to think of the costs of drugs, the time expended and the risks of treatment. It may be possible to draw up a financial balance sheet. Thus, if we are treating mild hypertension using the criteria of the MRC trial,[7] the costs of drugs and working time lost by 849 people who have to be treated in order to save one stroke are less than the cost of nursing the stroke that they would have got. The drugs used have side-effects but they are at least reversible, whereas a stroke is not.

Antenatal care is an example of a system of care deeply embedded in tradition. There is no question that it can save lives, but its traditional structure dates back to 1928 when an arbitrary plan was laid down which decided that women should be seen once a month from their 12th week of pregnancy, once a fortnight after 28 weeks, and then once a week for the last four weeks. The objectives were to monitor the mother's haemoglobin, blood pressure and urine. We now have to monitor the baby as well because if it is at risk in the uterus it can frequently survive outside the uterus in an intensive care unit. Sometimes it is necessary to do an amniocentesis.

The original schedule does not now make much sense. The

Figure 7.1 Should we start a clinic for a particular group of patients?

	Team	*Patient*
Advantages	Objectives of the session known so staff can start thinking along the right lines. Specialist staff and equipment.	May be seen more quickly. There may be specialist staff present, for example dietician for the diabetic clinic.
Disadvantages	Time has to be set aside, which reduces flexibility.	Sometimes patients have to miss work. Dislike of being seen in a clinic, especially family planning. Unable to raise other problems at the same time.

best time to know whether the baby is at risk from rhesus disease is as soon as the mother is pregnant. The ideal time to do an amniocentesis is about 15 weeks which is before the baby is too big to make a termination of pregnancy too harrowing. By writing down the objectives it is hoped that a more sensible strategy can be devised for the care of the patients.

2.   *Is it worth while having a separate clinic for a particular condition?* The easiest way to make a decision is to draw up a two-by-two table (see Figure 7.1) in which the boxes represent the advantages to the team and the disadvantages as against the advantages and disadvantages for the patient or client.

Thus, for hypertension, which does not require specialist staff or equipment, there are no advantages and a number of disadvantages. Suppose we were deciding to set up an antenatal clinic for the first time: one overwhelming advantage would be that the midwife and the doctor would meet over the patient and coordinate decisions, for instance, about where the woman should have her baby and how soon she should leave hospital. The woman herself could meet other women at the clinic which would enable her to make friends and share experience. The disadvantages are also less for her because she is entitled to time off work, and in any case women usually stop work towards the end of their pregnancy.

At the moment roughly one in five patients with diabetes goes to a hospital clinic (personal communication, SW Computer Users Group). This indicates that patients are fairly tolerant of clinics and it seems that starting clinics in general practice might benefit the rest of the patients and save some of the country's money.

3.   *Devising a note system or flow chart that will enable the objectives to be achieved*
Well laid out notes act as an *aide-mémoire* for the care of the patients. Because the obstetric record card has a series of columns that should be filled in at each attendance, failure to do something can be detected at a glance because there will be an empty space. The same principles can be applied to other diseases, for example a flow chart can be laid out as in Fig. 7.2. As can be seen in the chart it also helps to structure the clinic. The horizontal column designated N or D indicates whether it

Figure 7.2 Diabetic surveillance

Date	Smokes?	Seen optician Yes/No	Inspect Syringes	Feet	Weight	B.P.	Bl. Sugar Series	Acuity/ Fundoscopy	Medication a.m. p.m.
	N	N	N	N	N	N	N	D	D
	Always	Annually	6 mthly	6 mthly	6 mthly	Annually	Annually	Annually	Annually

Explanation
N = Nurse
D = Doctor

is the nurse or the doctor who is responsible for each phase of the clinic. Thus the patient goes to the nurse first, who discusses and deals with the items relevant to her. These include testing visual acuity, especially if the patient has not seen the optician, looking at the patient's feet and checking his or her syringes. Syringes are checked to make sure they are not worn out and to confirm that the patient is having the amount of insulin he or she claims to be having. When the nurse has done her measurements she can decide whether the doctor is likely to want to look at the fundi and if so can put in some Topicamide or other mydriatic drops. The patient then moves on to the doctor who can check the fundi and revise medication if that is needed.

4.   *Creation of a Morbidity Index*
A list of the patients with a particular disease enables the team to control their management and is an essential phase of the procedural review which they should do later on.

The morbidity index can also be used to check that patients have had at least the minimum standard of care laid down by the team protocol. For example, there are investigations which should be done at least annually. Thyrotoxic patients who have had radioactive iodine lapse into thyroid deficiency at about 10% a year, so these people should perhaps be checked regularly. Hypertensive patients are at risk of becoming uraemic so their blood urea levels should be checked regularly. Although yearly intervals for doing things are arbitrary it does have the administrative advantage that the check can be timed to coincide with the patient's birthday month.

The morbidity index can also be used when appointment lists are being made up, for instance, for diabetic clinics. Finally morbidity lists can be used for teaching.

5.   *Decision charts and clinical algorithms*
Many decisions have to be made when managing a group of patients with a chronic disease. Again some of these will be arbitrary. The decisions are necessary because much of the administration will be done by staff who have little clinical knowledge, or even by a computer which has none.

The simple way of designing an algorithm is to use a system of boxes. The boxes can be rectangles for straightforward

Figure 7.3   Protocol for the management of hypertension

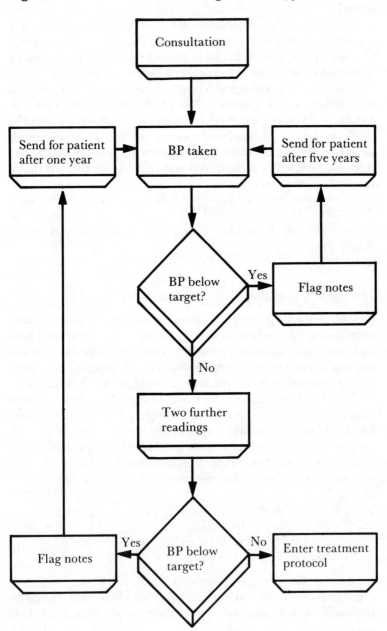

procedures that need doing and diamond shaped for decision points.

Suppose we take all patients in the practice and a decision is made to screen them for hypertension. The team decides that if the blood pressure level is below 149/99 mm Hg it can be reviewed in five years time. If, however, it is between 149/99 and 154/104 mm Hg it will have to be checked on at least three occasions to see if it drops below 149/99 mm Hg. If it does so the patient will be reviewed in five years, if not in one year. If, however, the blood pressure level is 155/105 mm Hg or above, and stays there after three readings, the patient will be entered into the treatment group. Writing this out in the form of a paragraph makes it difficult to comprehend but if it is set out in an algorithm it can look like Fig. 7.3. Designing such algorithms forces clear thinking and makes life a great deal easier later on. A number of algorithms are laid out in the appendix.

Emergency care and special procedures

As well as the long term management of chronic conditions the team has to be ready to deal with crises. The patient who goes into status asthmaticus may lose his or her life if he or she is not treated correctly and promptly.[8] The diabetic who goes hypoglycaemic may not die, but he could get brain damaged.

The reception staff have to know what to do, which partners to contact and what equipment he or she needs. If the practice has a nebuliser it has to be in working order and one individual, perhaps the practice nurse, must be made responsible for seeing that it is and that there is enough nebuliser solution in the box to treat the patient. This means check lists and instruction charts.

In the last chapter I pointed out one aspect of a dysfunctional team was that it ran by making many rigid rules. The same point can be made again. Written instructions must be kept to a minimum and must be relevant.

Practice Handbook

As the team takes on more tasks, so there will be more protocols. These will need regular review and are probably best kept in the form of a *practice handbook*. In a teaching practice the handbook can be reviewed whenever a new trainee arrives, perhaps by the trainer. Another suitable time to review it would be when the annual practice report is written.

Screening for disease

Screening for disease has been dealt with previously so it is necessary only to enumerate the important principles:

1. The disease is recognisable and there is an effective and agreed treatment for it.
2. A test is available for it that is both *specific* for the disease and *sensitive* enough to pick it up.
3. The test is not dangerous, nor too uncomfortable, nor too expensive.
4. The treatment is not too expensive.

When thinking about screening it is useful to decide how comprehensive the programme should be. Sometimes the yield of new cases can be greatly improved, i.e. the screening programme can be made a great deal more cost effective by selecting who will be screened. A classic example of this is testing the urine of new attenders at eye clinics to see if they have glycosuria and possibly then diabetes. This could be called category screening because it applies to a readily accessible subcategory of the population. In primary health care one category of patients who are comparatively easily checked and who are at a higher than average risk is the young women who come for oral contraceptive advice. They are almost by definition at risk of getting pregnant and many practices keep special record cards for them so that the practice can apply for contraceptive fees. These women can thus be more easily checked for rubella immunity either by doing their rubella titre or by making sure there is documented evidence of rubella inoculation.

Another way of looking at the benefits of a screening and prevention service is to calculate how much good could be done if the service was working completely effectively. Thus a general practitioner with an average sized list who ran a comprehensive service would expect to avoid:

- One rubella syndrome baby every 100 years

- One cancer cervix death every 12 years
- One cancer breast death every two years
- Ten to 12 premature deaths from cardiovascular disease every year

On this basis it could be argued that cardiovascular screening should take priority, except that we have to give considerable weight to the fact that, whereas cardiovascular morbidity is often due to self indulgence, the baby who gets the rubella syndrome has no choice at all.

References

1 Brown, G.W. and Harris, T. (1978) *Social origins of depression. A study of psychiatric disorder in women.* London: Tavistock Publications.
2 Van Hollie, T.B. (1986) Good news and bad news about obesity. *New. Engl. J. Med*, **314**; 239–40.
3 Armstrong, B.K. and Mann, J.I. (1985) Diet. In: Vessey, M.P., Gray, M. Eds. *Cancer, risks and prevention.* Oxford, Oxford University Press.
4 Stott, N.C.H. and Davis, C.H. (1979) The exceptional potential in each primary care consultation. *J. Royal Coll. Practitioners*, **29**; 201–5.
5 Tchobroutsky, G. (1978) Relation of diabetic control to the development of microvascular complications. *Diabetologia*, **15**; 143–52.
6 Engerman, R., Bloodworth, J.M.B. and Nelson, S. (1977) Relationship of microvascular disease in diabetes to metabolic control. *Diabetes*, **26**; 760–9.
7 Medical Research Council Working Party (1985) MRC trial of treatment of mild hypertension: principal results. *Br. Med. J.*, **291**; 97–104.
8 British Thoracic Association (1982) Death from Asthma in two regions in England. *Br. Med. J.*, **285**; 1251–5.

CHAPTER 8

Records

On the face of it, keeping medical notes needs no more than good handwriting and an ability to be methodical. In practice, the problems of medical recordkeeping occur mainly because the notes are expected to reconcile several opposing objectives.

Retrievability

Some information is of enormous importance. Often this information is not retrievable. If a patient had an operation which left a scar in the right iliac fossa but he did not have his appendix removed, clearly this should be prominently displayed in the notes and probably would be. Sometimes, however, the opposite occurs. An appendix is removed at the same time as a gynaecological operation is being done, and the fact is mentioned in the summary only in passing. If this information is forgotten it makes the subsequent diagnosis of an acute abdomen that bit more difficult.

Thus, in most cases, it is more important that information is retrievable than that the notes are comprehensive. This means that, when making notes, a judgement has to be made as to what to include. Display important information prominently e.g. 'anaphylactic reactions' on the front of the notes. Do not reiterate information that is readily available from the patient.

Notes shared by the team and separate sets of notes

The advantages of putting the notes of all the primary health care team members into the same folder are more theoretical than practical.

It could be argued that the health visitor's notes should be accessible to the doctor because if she has been weighing a child regularly and the child presents late on a Friday evening with diarrhoea he is going to need that information to decide whether the child is getting dehydrated. Similarly, if the practice nurse is taking out stitches she can look in the notes to see if the histology report has come through. On the other hand, the doctor usually knows where to look for the health visitor's records, and in any case mothers are often given their own card recording the baby's weight. In the same way, it does not take the practice nurse long to contact the receptionist or doctor to find out if the histology report is available.

If all documents are combined the notes may not always be available when they are needed. The baby comes to the health visitor's clinic but the health visitor cannot compare the previous weight and is irritated and frustrated that this is because the notes are with the secretary who is waiting for a letter to be dictated about them. It is worse still if a folder is lost or left in somebody's car while they go on holiday; none of the other professionals in the team has the information that he or she may need.

My own experience of an attempt to combine the health visitor's and the doctor's notes was abandoned because the combined record became too bulky, and the information was seldom of mutual interest. The principle of mutual access has, however, remained. Mutual access is not the same as combined notes.

There is no ideal system and there will always be problems such as embarrassment that could have been saved when the inevitable woman is invited by a nurse for a cervical smear and does not know herself that she has had a total hysterectomy.

Separate folders for chronic conditions

The exception to the general principle of different members of the health care team keeping separate notes is when two or more members of the team have frequent contact with the patient and when a large amount of information is collected. This particularly applies to patients attending the antenatal clinic and diabetic patients. There is much to be said for starting a separate A4 folder for each patient in such groups and indicating its existence by flagging the main notes so that the receptionists can make both sets of notes available whenever the patient consults. This is particularly useful in the case of the antenatal notes as the notes can then be made up at the first antenatal attendance and include the various forms that will be needed as times goes on. Forms such as Maternity Benefit Certificate (Mat B1) and others to remind staff to do a haemoglobin check at 28 or 36 weeks, or whenever the protocol demands.

Standardisation of records

There is a widespread belief that every piece of paper that enters the notes should be saved for ever in case it may be of interest in future legal proceedings. There is probably a good case to be made for keeping every item for a short time, but as soon as the notes reach a stage where important relevant clinical information is not easily found they are more likely to cause mistakes that can lead to legal proceedings. A decision should therefore be made about when to cull and what to throw out. Clearly the data that are duplicated need not be kept and there is probably little point in keeping material that has long since lost its relevance—for example, obstetric records of post-menopausal women, or the results of normal investigations done half-a-dozen years ago. The problem with this philosophy is that there is still a small possibility that a vital piece of information needed for litigation might be lost.

The first stage in the standardisation of records by teaching practices was the decision of the Joint Committee for Postgraduate Training in General Practice that the doctors' notes should be fixed in chronological order and that any correspondence or results of investigations should also be fixed in chronological order. Even this simple requirement resulted in considerable dismay, not least because of the amount of time and work involved. Many practices had decided on different systems already, such as filing all correspondence relevant to a chronic condition in one place. Sometimes individual partners had decided on a particular system which they were reluctant to abandon. The justification for the change was that it enabled a trainee to find his way about in the notes when he saw patients, thereby making it safer for the patient and not wasting the trainee's time. Some of the note-keeping systems that had to go had much to be said for them, however, and there was something lost in the new system. Nevertheless, once the system was working properly most doctors began to comment that they wondered how they had ever managed before.

As usual the problem is one of balancing flexibility against standardisation. Where standardisation is instituted it can be even more difficult to make subsequent changes, perhaps because people like to maintain the status quo.

The next phase in the standardisation of records by teaching practices is that teaching practice notes will have to contain a summary of every significant illness. This has forced people to think about what should be included and, more important, what should be left out.

Going back for a moment to the problem of throwing away notes that may have legal significance in years to come, the first point to make is that mistakes are less likely to occur if the notes are well laid out and orderly. Secondly, a doctor whose notes are chaotic is not going to be very credible if he is involved with the law. Thirdly, it is sometimes possible to predict when problems are going to occur and then more trouble can be taken to preserve the relevant old notes. If in doubt, keep them.

Cases where legal action is expected

Sometimes when patients are seen it can be predicted that there is going to be a legal involvement. When a man or woman states that he or she has been beaten up, the medical attendant is almost certain to be asked to give evidence about the injuries. The legal proceedings may be several years later; many women, for example, try to make a go of a marriage despite being physically assaulted again and again. This means that the notes have to be more comprehensive than usual as by the time they are needed it will be very difficult to remember what the injuries were.

- Record the time as well as the date when the patient was seen.
- Draw a sketch of the extent of the injuries, and if there are bruises record their colour.
- Record whether the bruises were compatible with the story given by the victim, and also record the victim's story.
- When rape is suspected the ideal person to carry out any examination is a police surgeon, who is often a woman. Police surgeons are specially trained and usually have equipment and containers to carry out a more thorough examination.

Who should have access to the data?

When data are confidential the fewer people who have access to them the less likely it is that there will be a breach of that confidentiality. The principle that doctors are liable for damages if they breach medical confidentiality is very long standing. Since September 1984 they have also been liable to pay compensation if patients suffer damage because of:
1. Loss of data
2. Destruction of the data without their (the doctors') consent
3. Disclosure of data
4. They are also liable (from May 1986) if the data are inaccurate and result in damage to the patients.

In the face of such penalties doctors may be reluctant to allow other members of the team to get at their notes. On the other hand, mutual trust is an essential element of team work and there will be many times when it will help the patient if he or she can be given information promptly.

What about the information given to the wrong person, or incorrect information being given to the right person? Giving information to the wrong person can happen very easily, as even telling a husband the result of his wife's pregnancy test is a breach of confidentiality. Incorrect information can be given even more easily. A blood test is taken and two investigations are done on it. The results of the first, say the haemoglobin concentration, may come back normal. This will be given to the patient over the telephone. When the result of the second one, say the thyroid function tests, comes in this may be abnormal, but the patient will not ring in again having already been told that his or her blood test is normal.

Hierarchy of access

The Data Protection Act gives rights of access by individuals to all automated information held on them. Thus if it is in computer file, or even a card index which can be mechanically or electronically accessed, they can see what is written and amend it. If the information is in any system such as a doctor's notes and letters, then they have no immediate legal right to see it. It does not, therefore, give them total access to their own medical records. Also under the same Act they have no right of access to data held on them by lawyers. The amount of access a patient will have to his or her medical records is still the subject of consultation and a decision has not yet been made by the Secretary of State. Meanwhile, there is a lot to be said for patients being given as much information as they want or feel they need. It is useful to know what operations they have had in the past and what immunisations. Much of this information is likely to be understood, so why should it not be given to them automatically? Indeed, they should be encouraged to hold such information themselves.

The next level of information in the notes relates to problems which have not yet been sorted out. The doctors may feel uncertain about what is going on and be trying to make a diagnosis. It is this uncertainty which would make the doctor feel unhappy about letting other people see what he has written.

Finally there is a layer of information that is genuinely relevant and which has been given in the strictest confidence. Information about sexual contacts in cases of venereal disease is an example. This information may not have come from the patient. A husband may be worried that he has infected his wife and may wish the doctor to put the information in the notes so that if she presents with symptoms suggesting an infection the doctor will be on the alert. Neither spouse may want this information thrust onto the wife.

Access to the notes by the patient

More important than being credible with the law is being credible with one's patients and clients. Some patients are asking to see their notes, and others are being shown them routinely by their doctors. The Data Protection Act enables people to find out if their names are on registers and if they are, to see and correct facts in those registers. Access by patients to their notes is a logical extension of this principle. There has been widespread support from doctors for this and, although some of the less complimentary remarks that used to be written in the notes by exasperated doctors and others will become less frequent, the change will lead to more openness and perhaps to less dependence.

Allowing the patients to see the notes when they wish reassures them that there is nothing to hide. It also gives them a

Table 8.1 Advantages and disadvantages of patients seeing their own records

Advantages	*Disadvantages*
Patients have a right to know what has been said about them.	The patient may not understand the terminology used and may be frightened or misled.
Patients need access to the data in order to make decisions about themselves.	Data in medical notes are often opinion rather than facts. The patient may not appreciate this.
Accuracy is improved if patients check the records.	There may be privileged information in the notes, for example, from a spouse.
	Open access may push the doctor towards defensive medicine, which is usually not in the patient's interests.
	Medical records are also about the doctor who makes them. He may wish to have *aides-mémoire* to help him in his problem solving. This information is his property and not the patient's. He may have a right not to disclose it. Doctors should have a right to prune such information from the notes before open access becomes law.

chance to correct errors. There may be problems all the same— for example, there is always the possibility that the patient will see information relating to a third party which, as has already been said, constitutes a breach of confidentiality.

If a patient asks to see his or her own notes and is refused he or she is likely to become hostile and feel his or her worst suspicions may be confirmed. The most sensible line to take is to explore what the reason is for the request and then to stay with the patient when he or she is reading through them. If there is extensive correspondence from another person, say a doctor or social worker, his or her permission may need to be sought before his or her letters can be read.

CHAPTER 9

Performance Review

Performance review is the name given to the process of comparing what the team is trying to achieve with what it has actually achieved. This has been called medical audit, but as the word audit has so many bad connotations and in itself was derived from the latin 'audere', meaning to hear, which is not what takes place, the term 'performance review' was coined. aim of performance review is to see how well the team is doing, and how they are performing.

Why do performance review?

The why of performance review is bound up with the concept of accountability. An old-fashioned distinction between a profession and a trade was that people did not follow a profession simply for profit, but also out of altruism. A profession also required a period of learning and this meant that the public had to take the advice of professionals on trust as only by acquiring the learning themselves could they check directly that they were getting what they paid for. This attitude still persists and is also associated with members of the professions receiving higher status and, in some cases (doctors perhaps but not the nurses), higher pay.

Clearly, if a professional group depends on public trust it is in its own interests to police itself and make sure that as a whole it is worthy of that trust. This used to be achieved by not allowing doctors to enter the profession until they had passed certain examinations and got over hurdles that showed they had sufficient skills and knowledge to do the job. The situation is now changing so rapidly that having the skills and knowledge is not sufficient. Somehow or other doctors and others have got to start showing that they not only can do the job, but that they actually are doing it. The responsibility of the general practitioner is not just to the individual patient but to all the patients on his list. He is paid as much to look after those patients who do not come to see him as he is for those who do. Failure in this task will result in the general public imposing a system of performance review. In some cases the government has already started to do this—for example, family practitioner committees are refusing to reimburse rents for premises if they think the premises are inadequate.

Some would argue that as the government pays the bill it might as well be left to the government to monitor the standards, just as in a capitalist society people should be allowed to pay for the medicine they think they want rather than the medicine they need. The implication is that to give people what the doctor thinks they need is for them to be patronised. In the long term this may be right, but medicine changes fast and it is too complicated to be run by external audit. Thus, under the present system of reimbursement for screening for cervical cancer, doctors are paid to do smears every five years, whereas many doctors believe that for the campaign to be effective three years would be more appropriate.[1] The medical profession would lose much status if it allowed medical services to be controlled by others.

Many doctors regard their personal freedom to prescribe what they wish as the linchpin of the doctor–patient relationship. Doctors and other medical staff have a duty to provide the best that they can for a patient under their care, but when resources are limited giving something to one patient may deprive another. Doctors therefore have a moral duty to see that resources are not wasted, and that they are actually achieving what they set out to achieve.

How to do performance review

The technique for performance review has now been worked out. It is the systematic setting of standards, the collection of data to see if those standards have been achieved, and the appropriate change either of standards or the methods used to try to achieve them. This cycle is then repeated.

Performance review is not about scientific research. It is not something that is done once and then abandoned. It is, or should be, an integral part of long term management.[2]

Stages of performance review (medical audit)
1. Standards agreed
2. Data collected
3. Data compared with agreed standard
4. Appropriate change made
5. Go to 1 where new standards may be set.

Setting the standards

The standards for performance review have to be thought about carefully. On the one hand they must not be so low as to be absurd, and on the other hand they must be low enough to be a realistic target. A simple rule is to ask people who are going to do an audit what they *think* they are currently achieving. For example, how often do the district nurse and the general practitioner think they review together the care of a patient whom they are both looking after? Are patients being offered an appointment to see the doctor of their choice within a reasonable period of time? How frequently are adult patients getting their blood pressure taken?

The experience of most people who undertake performance review is that their actual performance is shatteringly lower than what they would have predicted. I had thought that I would know whether my patients with asthma smoked cigarettes, but when I came to check it many of them had never been asked, and some of the patients had not been seen for over a year. Standards may be described as *normative* or *criterion* based.

Normative standards are those derived from other people – from everybody's performance. In other words how near the normal is a particular team or practitioner. There are several problems with normative standards. Firstly because a particular team is about average it does not mean that it is doing well, indeed one could say that almost by definition it could do better. How could it do better? Take outpatient referrals to a Psychiatrist. Suppose these were higher than average it could be argued that all patients who could benefit from psychiatric treatment were more likely to receive it. On the other hand some patients could have been referred unnecessarily, thereby wasting resources and perhaps causing unnecessary distress.

This particular example can be taken one step further. It is assumed that if information about performance is fed back to people they will adjust their performance towards the norm. The trouble is that some may use inappropriate methods of adjusting towards the norm. A low referring practitioner who is told that he is below average may begin to refer more patients but they will not necessarily be those who will benefit from referral.

Normative standards are often used by external agencies such as the prescription pricing bureau who look at the costs of every doctor prescribing and then interview those who spend most. Many practices collect data on such things as referral and visiting rates. When they do this they may have an underlying assumption that they are doing an audit and that their standards are normative. They quickly find out the problems about normative standards, and that may be the most valuable part of the exercise. The data has however got a separate use which is that it enables the team to plan the use of their time more effectively.

Criterion based performance review is when standards are generated from within the group. Here the problem is to make them sensible and relevant. Compare, for example, two criterion based audits. One practice decides that as a minimum standard a doctor should be present at all deliveries; another decides that all women presenting for advice on birth control should have documentation in the notes of either a rubella titre or a rubella injection. There is plenty of room for nit picking with both sets of criteria. How often will the doctor be doing anything useful at the delivery in a GP unit? And, if there are times when, because of the speed of the second stage of labour, he is physically unable to get there, surely the midwife should be sufficiently well trained to manage neonatal resuscitation in his absence? With the rubella criteria it could be argued that it is difficult enough for a young woman to come for advice, and any fear of an injection or venepuncture is just one more thing to put her off. In any case, how useful is a low titre in somebody who thinks she has had an injection for rubella?

Collection of data

Make the collection of data easy and it is more likely that it will be complete. It is not just a question of assembling information, but also one of making the information readily accessible so that progress can be monitored and adjustments made. If possible the results should be set out in the form of histograms, ideally with colours. Here again, thinking it through before starting is well worthwhile.

> A practice decides to screen all adults for hypertension. A receptionist goes through each set of notes to see if a normal, as defined in the criteria, blood pressure has been recorded recently. If it has she puts, say, a green flag in the notes (in this case a piece of card which protrudes above the Lloyd George folder). Where a blood pressure is yet to be taken a red flag is used, and a yellow one if the patient is a known hypertensive. A glance along the filing shelves will give an immediate idea of the progress the practice is making: at first there will be mainly red stickers; eventually it is hoped the stickers will be entirely green and yellow. It is also then relatively easy to generate a histogram.

Appropriate change

The only thing that can be predicted about performance review is that as data are collected there is likely to be a change in the standards that were originally set, or in the ways in which they are to be achieved. This is an aim of performance review and when audits are described in journals it is surprising how little emphasis is given to it.

> A practice decided to check the rubella status of women coming for birth control advice. As patients were seen the receptionist flagged the notes of any who had not met the criteria laid down. As no woman was given more than six months' supply of the pill, and all of them should have come back after one year for coil or cap checks, it was assumed that after 18 months the majority would have been seen and the rubella status of the cohort would be known, those who had no record in their notes of rubella immunity would be offered a rubella titre and, if that was negative, an injection.
>
> A register of all women receiving birth control advice was kept on a computer, so it was relatively easy to keep an account of progress. After 18 months only a quarter of the women's rubella status was known and a meeting was held to discuss the

disappointing result. The doctors identified the problem as lack of time in the consultation, where they were taking on too much in the way of opportunistic health education. There was also a problem because if another investigation was to be offered to the patient, much time would be taken up in explanation and discussion.

The senior receptionist had been enthusiastic about the project and to some extent had taken it under her own wing. She felt able to explain what was needed to the patients, especially if she could give them a handout. It was therefore agreed that the receptionists should take a much more positive role, looking out for notes of patients whose rubella status was not known and broaching the subject when these patients arrived for their appointments.

This particular audit illustrated a number of points to the partners. First, that useful data could be generated quite easily. Secondly, that when the data had been collected they felt in a much better position to make realistic decisions. In fact they realised that good decisions cannot be made without information. Thirdly, they realised that the doctor is always stressed when consulting and that the more work that is put on to him or her the less likely it is to get done. This particular practice did not have, and still has not got, its full quota of ancillary staff.

Different types of performance review

Performance review has been classified as either *internal*, that is to say performed by the team on itself, or *external*. An internal audit has just been described and it has many strengths. It teaches the team something about themselves and is more likely to be completed because it is something they decide to do themselves. In doing it they are taking responsibility for their own standards and performance.

An *external* performance review (or audit) is done by somebody from outside the team. It thus carries the implication that standards are being checked and that people may be taken to task for failing to achieve suitable levels. On the other hand, external audits have great strengths. It is often difficult to see yourself from the outside. Sometimes by getting other people to come and have a look the team will be stimulated to start thinking more carefully about their aims.

Peer review is a key concept in the new quality of care

initiative by the Royal College of General Practitioners. It is proposed that College members formally visit each other's practices to study how well they are doing. It is also suggested that Fellowship of the College should be given only to those who apply for it and who submit themselves to a practice inspection.

There is, of course, the semantic difficulty that peer review by the College of General Practitioners is just internal audit one step further up the chain.

Structure, Process, Outcome

Performance review can examine many aspects of the work of the primary health care team and it is convenient to classify these under the headings Structure, Process and Outcome. Notice that these are not all-embracing; performance review cannot, for example, examine attitudes of the staff towards the patients.

Structure means the physical objects involved in patient care, specifically such things as notes and equipment. Standards can be set for the notes, such as whether they contain proper summaries. Data can be collected on the state of the notes and so on.

Process refers to what is going on. What are the standards set for the appointments system? Are they being met?

Outcome refers to results achieved and is more difficult to apply in a primary health care setting because many of the results are at one or more removes. Thus deaths are relatively rare. It could perhaps be worth looking at the outcome for obesity clinics or smoking cessation clinics. In many cases patients relapse!

References

1 IARC Working group on Evaluation of Cervical Cancer Screening Programmes (1986) Screening for squamous cervical cancer: duration of low risk after negative results of cervical cytology and its implications for screening policies. *B. Med. J.*, **293**; 659–64.
2 Shaw, C.D. (1980) Aspects of audit. *B. Med. J.*, **280**; 1256–8, 1314–6, 1361–6, 1443–6.

CHAPTER 10

The Caring Personality – People in Their Professional Roles

This chapter is about the underlying, usually unspoken, problems of caring professionals in resolving the conflicts between altruism and the need to make a livelihood. The dilemmas are not new, nor are the answers clear cut. The aim of this chapter is to discuss the sort of difficulties people may have in their roles in the team, in the hope that by thinking about what they do they may be able to make constructive changes in the way they work.

First, it is probably worth exploring some of the conflicts in the National Health Service by looking at some of the contradictory underlying assumptions.

1. The caring professions grew up out of the church which was a charitable foundation. Therefore the only people who should go into the caring professions are those who like people, or indeed love them.
2. Resources are limited and the job of the primary health care worker is to help ration them.
3. People are divided into those who are sick and those who are healthy. In some cases where there is doubt the doctor decides which category they fall into. Sick people have an obligation to try to get better, specifically by obeying the instructions of the medical attendants. (Incidentally, people who have to obey usually have inferior status.)
4. Some primary health care professionals undergo long training. They also carry much responsibility. They should therefore be well paid. On the other hand, they will get rewards from the job, so that perhaps they should not be paid at all.
5. The public pay for the health service through taxes. They

therefore have a right to the best service available, delivered promptly.

There are many other assumptions about the delivery of medical care, and most people who work in the National Health Service would agree that there is a lot of truth in the ones that I have already produced. The trouble is that many of them cannot be resolved with each other.

Take, for example, the question of preventive medicine. If a woman is offered a cervical smear test and decides not to have it, most people would agree that it is her business, although now there is evidence that cervical cancer is a venereal disease some would argue that it is her husband's business as well. On the other hand, if abnormality is discovered early enough it may save her life. This affects not just her but also any young children she may have. The children may be affected in both the short and long term as there is evidence that childhood bereavement can predispose to depression in later life.[1] Clearly it would be better if she had a smear test, in the same way as it would be better if she did not smoke in pregnancy and did breast-feed her baby. Therefore it is the job of the primary health care team to persuade her about these things, especially as once she has been diagnosed as having cancer she will expect the wheels to turn fast and expensively to get her cured.

Primary health care workers are particularly vulnerable in this sort of situation. Unlike, say, the radiotherapy specialists or the gynaecologists, they are in a position where theoretically they could have avoided the problem, and in the end it will be for them to pick up the pieces, both physical and emotional.

Professionalism

It is part of the job of primary health care workers to have to cope with these dilemmas and to do their best to allocate their time and resources in what they see to be the most effective way possible. This means looking at problems in both the long and short terms.

It may be possible to draw up a balance sheet of the costs in terms of time and resources spent and the benefit obtained—for example, comparing the costs, on the one hand, of screening the population for hypertension and treating cases that have been identified with the cheapest available drugs, with, on the other hand, the costs in terms of hospital beds, nursing time and so on of caring for patients who have had no treatment and have sustained a stroke.

Usually, however, the basic information is not available. For example, for how long do patients who have had a stroke need to be in hospital? In any case, how do you compare such disparate activities as spending time with the bereaved and advising mothers about their children's diets to stop them becoming obese?

It is a characteristic of primary health care that there is much uncertainty. In other branches of care and other jobs many rules are made to help people make decisions. Learning to cope with uncertainty and to allocate time and resources on the basis of inadequate data is one of the professional skills of the primary health care worker. It is something he or she has to learn to do.

Arising out of this is another problem: deciding where the limits of responsibility lie. Where the job is undefined and time is limited just how much should be devoted to any particular task and which tasks should be left undone? One way people used to solve this problem was by declaring themselves overwhelmed with work. This meant that they would be far too busy to spend time thinking it through and just get on with what came immediately to hand. Two categories would inevitably get the most time: those who shouted loudest—that is, patients who learnt the trick of attracting attention, perhaps by insisting on their rights, or by sheer persistence—and those whose problems were pleasant and easy to treat, such as young women with children or people needing contraceptive advice. Neither of these two categories is the most deserving. It is therefore a necessary part of professionalism to be organised and not to be overwhelmed.

There is also the question of limited returns for work put in. To go back to the women who do not answer several letters asking them to come for cervical smears: a study on these women was done by visiting them in their homes and interviewing them. The aim of the study was to find out why they had not responded to two offers of screening. It was done by a young woman doctor who asked about their reaction to the requests in as informal a way as she could. She had no problems getting all the people visited to see her and to talk to her about their reason for not coming. It turned out that many of them regarded cancer with a certain amount of superstition and, just as country people in England do not like seeing single magpies, so they felt that thinking about or mentioning cancer might bring it on (personal communication, Bailey, G.). Inevitably they wanted nothing to do with cervical smears. Most of these women were conventional, somewhat timid people who were probably not at high risk and it was clear that it would require much effort and tact to get them to come in. For instance, this personal approach by a friendly woman doctor did not result in a single peson taking up the offer for a cancer smear.

Power Bases and Paymasters

Although most members of the team work from the same building not all of them regard it as their primary base. The district nurse may take messages in the practice premises and from the central nurses administrative office. The health visitors may spend much of their time working from the practice premises, yet they are responsible to the District Nursing Officer, who will ask them to come to meetings and expect them to pursue policies that she or he decides on.

Inevitably this results in a split in loyalties, and the problem is to identify where the pressure is coming from. What can happen is that groups outside the primary health care team— for example, the obstetric authorities—feel obliged to try to raise standards in the community. The simplest method is to collect data and compare different primary health care centres to see how well they are doing. Questions can be asked about the details of obstetric care, how many attend parentcraft classes and so on. The intention is to stimulate the midwife to do better. Some of the tasks may be outside the midwife's control. This puts her in the difficult position of having to denigrate either the superiors who employ her or the team. Unless she has some insight into the situation only chance will decide which group she will support, or perhaps her own personal view as to whether the targets set are realistic and worth while.

If she does not think they are worth while she can always try to persuade the people who are trying to push them through, or at least she should discuss them. If she does think they are worth while she is more likely to succeed in achieving them if she does not get angry with those who are frustrating her.

Exploitation of the Job to Serve Personal Needs

Dealing with the sick is an emotional experience. Inevitably there will be much pain, discomfort and distress. Those who look after ill people will feel needed, indeed wanted. What sort of person takes on this role?

Judging by the effect it has, many of them have severe problems of their own.[2] The suicide rate among doctors is twice that of the rest of the population and there are many other indications of underlying problems including such things as marriage breakdown and alcoholism.

It is possible that people who have problems are attracted to caring professions in the hope of attracting some of the emotional warmth that they themselves missed in childhood.

Transactional analysis has proposed an attractive theory as to how this can be achieved. Basically it professes that there are three ego states. The three ego states are the parent, the adult and the child.[3] An ego state is a system of 'thinking, feeling and behaving'.

Sometimes we think, feel and behave like rational adults, on other occasions like small children. We like to think that we behave most of the time like adults, especially in our professional lives, and by this we mean being the rational sensible person that we have come to think of as an appropriate person to be in a responsible job. It seems we learn these values from our own parents who spent much time and effort giving us signals as to what was, in their view, adult behaviour. Unfortunately the child-like ego state persists and also needs to find ways of expressing itself.

Many health care professionals have had an abnormal childhood in which, for one reason or another, the child-like ego state has been blocked. This means that they can behave like adults and parents controlling others, but the need to act out the child is blocked and only their parents can act as surrogates for the child in the carer. Thus a patient can be greedy and demanding or whatever, but the carer remains upright and controlled like a parent ready to help.

The ability to tolerate all these emotions in others is useful in the short term because many of the situations that occur in everyday life also occur in the primary health care setting. Many clients or patients want somebody to lean on during a crisis. In the long term the carer may be overwhelmed and may either breakdown because his or her own personal needs are not being met, or become so disillusioned that he or she starts to behave destructively. Even when he or she does not do this there is a danger of the patients becoming dependent, something which is not what is wanted if the role of the primary health care team is to foster autonomy.

References

1 Brown, G.W. and Harris, T. (1978) *Social origins of depression*. London, Tavistock Publications.
2 Rose, K.D. and Rostow, I. (1973) Physicians who kill themselves. *Arch. Gen. Psychiatry*, **29**; 800–5.
3 Berne, E. (1964) Games people play, A. Deutsch. Now in Penguin books.

CHAPTER 11

The Case Conference

The case conference is a powerful technique that has crept into the repertoire of primary health care almost, it seems, by chance. The case conference is a formal meeting that differs from a committee or management meeting in that it is often a one-off affair. It also differs in usually having no formal agenda and in the rules governing it being different, although in some ways just as definite.

The case conference usually relates to a person or a family. It can be called by any member of the team, but the essential qualification for being able to call one is that those who do so have direct responsibility for the client and usually first hand contact.

Which clients are suitable for a case conference?

In a well run primary health care team much emphasis is put on communication, especially informal communication. This is adequate when only two or three people are involved and when the situation is moving slowly.

Informal communication cannot cope when more than three or four people are involved, especially if those people come from very widely differing disciplines. Sometimes the carers do not realise how many other agencies the client is drawing on and, sometimes, an apparently stable situation can suddenly boil over after a comparatively minor incident, such as a bout of illness or an accident.

An example

Case History

Miss Mary H aged 79 had always been somewhat eccentric but had coped well. She had been to university but had never used her degree. She was well off, indeed her solicitor felt that she was one of his most astute clients in the handling of her investments. She lived in an old person's flat where there was a resident warden, and she rarely saw her doctor. On several of the few occasions when she did see him she confided to him that in her opinion most of the problems in the West were due to the 'Soviets' influencing events by using the 'airwaves'. She had perhaps become more unkempt as the years went by and more obsessed with her bowels.

The situation changed abruptly when the warden discovered that Miss H had had a summons to go to court. Apparently she had scraped another car while out driving but had not stopped. When challenged she denied that she had been in an accident and said that the damage to her own car was just a scrape which everyone else was making an excessive fuss about. It was soon discovered that this was but one of a series of accidents and that her insurance company had refused her further cover.

A social worker had been asked to visit because neighbours had seen her every evening standing in her front window staring East to make sure the moon came up. There were complaints because the house smelt and this was tracked down to food left uneaten for several weeks in a cupboard. A pet puppy was left to die of heat exhaustion in the back of her car. The home-help service arranged for the flat to be cleaned up. Miss H then accused them of stealing her property as after the clean up she said she could not find anything.

The case conference was called by the head of the home help service and was held at the medical centre. It included the warden, the psychiatric social worker, a representative of the police and her doctor. Much new information was added, including the detail that her garage mechanic had guessed what was going on and had managed to keep her off the road for some time by making sure the car would not start. The police force had been extraordinarily tolerant and had on several occasions escorted her home.

It was decided at the case conference that she had become too much of a danger to herself and the public and that urgent admission to a mental hospital was needed. It was felt that both the police and the garage mechanic were, strictly speaking, acting outside the law, and that the old lady might anyway buy herself a new car, something she could easily afford to do.

The doctor was asked to contact the local psychiatrist who had special responsibility for the elderly and admission to a mental hospital under an Order was then arranged.

Arranging a Case Conference

Who calls it

Any member of the team can arrange a case conference and should do so as soon as they realise that too many people are involved for effective care to go without them talking to each other. In the case of Miss H the home-help superintendent knew that many people had seen Miss H but did not know how much they knew about what was going on or even at what stage they had become involved. The psychiatric social worker had visited in the past but could not remember when she had first become involved.

Most case conferences are called by social workers. This is partly because they have legal obligations towards their clients, especially under the Mental Health Act. In such cases they are often involved with other carers.

How to call it

Whoever decides to call a case conference has to telephone those they know who are involved to discover if they wish to come and what times would suit them. The people they are contacting may know of others who may be involved. A case conference can flounder because a key person has not been invited: if the problem is to do with housing, for example, a representative from the housing department would make all the difference.

It does not matter where they meet provided there is sufficient space and a chair for everybody. From time to time the patient herself, or if it is a child, his or her parents, are invited. This would be unusual if it is a first meeting.

Protocol of a Case Conference

A case conference needs a chairman. As the participants are of equal status there is no reason why any particular person should be in the chair, except that the person who called the case conference is likely by now to have the most information. Having said this, whatever the situation, the conference must open with a formal agreement on who is to be in the chair. Sometimes when there is an important legal issue the social worker will invite the head of his department to chair a conference that he himself has called.

Once the chairman has been decided he or she can start by outlining the situation from his or her own point of view. Each member of the conference is then asked in turn to give his or her version. This means that the person who called the conference and who is likely to start the proceedings should have the case history clearly set out, perhaps at some length. He or she may need to read it out, although on the whole it is better not to. Everybody else should also have brought their own notes, so that factual details can be corrected or confirmed. Errors of fact can be corrected after each person has given his account, but that is all that can be done. General discussion must wait until everybody has finished.

It seems that people often respond to others in a pattern, perhaps as a result of a childhood experience. This pattern transfers itself to the carers, depending on the role in which they have been cast. Thus a particular agency may have been seen as authoritarian and not trustworthy since childhood. For example, the police service may fall into this role and the pattern will persist through life. Another agency may have the reverse image so that, for example, the doctor may be seen as the only stable person. These sort of patterns will emerge as each participant at the case conference says their bit. The other participants will then be able to build up a more complete picture of their client as they hear what the others have to say. They will also learn something about the attitudes of the other people at the conference, what their priorities are, how caring they are, and what they see as their own limitations.

The next phase is one of discussion. No decisions have to be taken but views can be exchanged. As no concrete proposal may have yet been made this phase of the case conference is more like a buzz group than a committee meeting.

In due course, certain issues may emerge about the client or his family, such as who is at risk and who is being most manipulative. If nobody is particularly at risk the case conference may reach a collective decision to do nothing. Otherwise individuals may accept responsibility for taking particular courses of action.

Making a Decision at a Case Conference

Although it is theoretically possible for a chairman to change a case conference to a committee meeting by asking people to propose and second motions on what should be done and then taking a vote, this is seldom necessary in practice. A case conference usually develops like a group discussion, with the problem being discussed until a consensus is reached or at least until it becomes clear that no consensus will be reached in the time available.

Ending the Case Conference

As the case conference comes to an end the chairman will have to start drawing out the most important points and confirming any commitments the different participants may have made. For example, in the case of Miss H the police representative agreed that their previous rather conciliatory approach of helping her to drive home when seen out in a car was no longer appropriate as it simply colluded with her attitude that nothing serious had occurred and that driving while not insured was an unimportant detail. Equally, the doctor was to make sure that she was to be seen promptly by the psychiatrist.

Finally the chairman has to make arrangements for follow-up. Usually this entails no more than letting those present have a synopsis of what has occurred, but sometimes a date for another meeting has to be found.

Further Reading

Campbell, Alistair V. and Higgs, R. (1982) In that case: Medical ethics in everyday practice. *Darton, Longman and Todd.*

This book is well worth reading as a whole but the chapter on the Case Conference has many useful highlights.

CHAPTER 12

Patient Participation

There is increasing realisation in all the public services that a take it or leave it attitude is no longer good enough. People realise that their health service, just like their schools and their police force, costs them money and is there to serve them. The health service has been one of the last public services to start looking for feedback from the people it is there to serve. Apart from a few pioneering general practices the primary health care workers are probably behind the rest.

Most doctors probably feel that they give an excellent service already. Many patients probably feel the same way, except that there are always stories going round of indifferent or offhand treatment of people by receptionists, hurried doctors and unfeeling staff. If the health service were a commercial enterprise theoretically the general public could influence it at their point of contact with it simply by refusing to use services that could be bought elsewhere. Where the service is publicly owned the patient can lose this basic right. A patient participation group does not give the patients total control, but it at least gives them a voice.

A patient participation group can provide:

- Consumers' views and opinions
- Suggestions for improvements in buildings and services
- Resources: expert advice; practical help; money from fund raising.

Consumers' views and opinions

There is always a risk that the people who select themselves to be the spokes-men and women for their community will not be typical of those they represent. They tend to be either the more active or the most talkative. It is therefore important that any committee is as representative as possible; special care must be taken to draw from the most vulnerable groups such as the elderly, women with young children, the physically handicapped and even the housebound.

The participation group will know something about how good the services provided are because they have to use them. They will also have learnt about the weaknesses in the system just by sitting in the waiting room and chatting to other patients. When a participation group committee wants to collect ideas and opinions it can actually have members sitting in the waiting room with the aim of talking to other patients and getting their views.

It is part of the function of a particiption group to edit complaints into constructive suggestions. Sometimes questionnaires may be needed or a complaints box. These can be given out in the waiting room or sent out to patients. Clearly the participation group could not be given a list of patients registered with the practice as this would be a breach of confidentiality, but there is no reason why the questionnaire should not be mailed by the practice staff.

Another way of getting information is to hold meetings to collect opinions.

Suggestions for improvements

The relationship between the patient participation group and the primary health care team is complicated by the doctors having independent contractor status and often owning the premises. This limits what can be done in the way of making structural alterations and it also means that if money is raised for equipment the ownership of that equipment has to be clearly set out. At the same time, the patient participation group can do a great deal that the partners cannot do because of their vested interests. For example, the patients can lobby the council for alterations in car parking arrangements, or access roads. Some primary health care teams have found members of participation groups with special skills which they are willing to use for the benefit of the medical centre. For example, when people who are artistic do cartoons for practice leaflets or posters.

Some suggestions may be for things that do not involve much

in the way of resources, such as a change in the timing of surgeries or clinics.

Resources

The most important resources that the patient participation group can tap are time and energy. It seems that there is considerable goodwill in the community and a desire to do something for others. At one extreme it may extend to organising vast charity events to raise big sums of money; at the other it may mean giving a few hours every now and again to help weigh babies in the clinic or to sit with an elderly person.

Expertise is normally not so much expensive as difficult to find. Many people from all sorts of backgrounds come into the primary health care premises every week. They may well be experts in their own field and may spot things which could be done better, but feel reluctant to offer gratuitous advice. A patient participation group is one way they can offer suggestions without risking a rebuff. Sometimes a patient participation group will wish to make a formal proposal for some change and will need their own members to advise them on what is practical. For example, a knowledge of local government machinery could help if an approach was being made to improve car parking facilities.

Meetings

The usual pattern for a patient participation group is to have open meetings—for example, talks or lectures on health which are held in any suitable building, including the health centre—and committee meetings, which are always on the committee's own ground, for instance in somebody's house.

From the start it has to be made clear that the professional staff of the primary health care team will come to these meetings only by invitation. This is not just because there may be complaints about the staff which have to be dealt with. It is because the patient participation group has to retain its independence.

A good patient participation group can address many issues that used to be thought of as the business of the doctors alone.

For example, one group heard that a new partner was to be appointed and was able to tell the existing partners of their preference for a woman doctor.

Getting started

A founding committee has to be formed. The first stage is to identify people who would be willing to serve on such a committee by leaving out leaflets in the waiting room or by attaching them to repeat prescriptions. An inaugural meeting can then be held at which the officers of the committee can be chosen and the constitution and procedures drawn up. The aims of the association should be agreed; how often and where there should be meetings, who should be on the committee, and how long they should remain in office. Decisions also have to be made about funds, whether there should be a subscription, how large it should be and so on.

Further Reading

Petrie, J. (1986) Publicising patient participation groups. *Br. Med. J.*, **293**; 369–70.
Pritchard, P.M. (1980) Patient participation in general practice. *R. Coll. Gen. Pract.*, Occasional Paper 17.

CHAPTER 13

Computers in Primary Health Care

Although in theoretical terms a computer cannot do anything that cannot be done manually, in practical terms computerisation adds much to the ability of the primary health care team. The time between the conception of a new technique in primary health care and its use in the majority of teams is dramatically shortened. An illustration of this is the age–sex register. In the mid-1960s a progressive practice would have an age–sex register which would be used mainly for the interest of the partners and as a teaching tool. It took another 10 years for it to be used for checking developmental screening and cervical smears, and then only in the most enthusiastic practices. We have now reached the stage where a practice can install a computer for a few thousand pounds and can immediately move on to doing recalls, follow-ups, performance reviews and carefully monitored repeat prescribing. Theoretically a good software development for one system can be translated so it works for every other system, and so management can be improved rapidly across the board. New ideas that in the past took 20 years to implement will soon take only a year or two to become common practice.

Already microcomputers are so cheap that partnerships are no longer asking themselves *if* they should start but *when* they can start. The computer will earn them money by helping them call up more of their patients who need services, such as cervical smears, for which the doctors will get paid. This helps with the costs but it is unlikely to make much of a profit. What it does is to improve the service.

Increased staff

One of the ironies of computers is that instead of saving staff and paper they often increase both. Although this can happen because unnecessary tasks are being done in a primary health care setting it is more likely that it is because the computer makes it possible to do many things which were impossible with a manual system. For example a comprehensive cervical smear campaign can be set up. This makes more work for the practice nurse but it also makes more work for the reception staff because even if the letters offering appointments are written by the computer, the staff still have to allocate extra appointments, supervise and support patients coming along for their smears. They then have to inform them of the results and there is also extra work dealing with abnormal smears.

The effectiveness of the computer depends on the software which now constitutes much of the cost. There are several systems available but at least one large software firm has dropped out of primary health care computing. Some software has been written by the GPs themselves; it varies from relatively simple systems which handle repeat prescribing to some much more sophisticated programs that are able to monitor a wide range of team activities. Nevertheless the situation at the moment is that most software is written by people who are not primary health care workers and who therefore do not fully understand all the problems. This can lead to feelings of vulnerability for the users, which can only be overcome by their trying to understand the equipment and its limitations. They also have to feed the problems back to software firms so that programs can be modified.

Installing a computer

Effect on the office staff

The main burden of installing a computer usually falls on the receptionists. They have to learn how to work the system and have to adapt themselves to a mixed system of electronic and manual record keeping. Where Family Practitioner Committees are computerised, practice registers can be downloaded onto the practice computer with little effort. This has much reduced the time and work needed to get a practice computer system working. It does, however, mean that the office staff now have to learn how to use the machine before

Figure 13.1   Uses of the computer in a primary health care setting

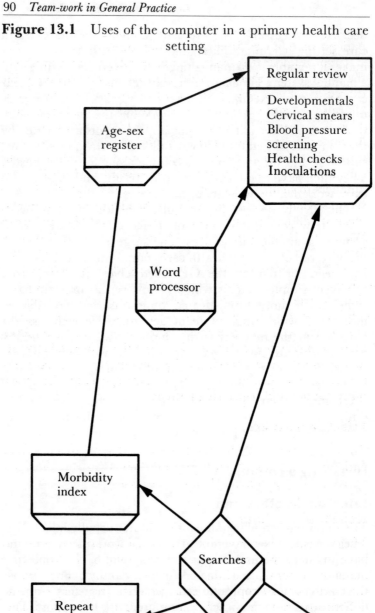

starting whereas they used to be able to use the phase of putting patients on to the register as an apprenticeship.

Unfortunately it is easy to misunderstand some aspects of the program and thereby create a lot of work for the future. For example one popular piece of software has the facility of allocating identification numbers to certain groups of patients. This is a form of electronic flagging. It has many uses, for instance a partner with a particular interest may want to follow up a group of patients. Another may want to track patients who can earn the practice fees. It is easy to allocate the identification numbers to such groups of patients but unless a good system is set up so that everyone knows what the identification numbers mean it will not be used, and the follow up will be inefficient. Worse still the meaning of the identification numbers can be forgotten.

At first the office staff may have difficulty in dropping manual systems that they know and trust. They have to learn that electronic systems are a waste of time if they insist on duplicating everything manually. Fortunately they quickly realise that whatever deficiencies there may be in a computer, there are many fewer than on the manual register and they are much more easily checked. The computer will save the reception staff time in several areas, but especially with repeat prescriptions and registering patients.

Effect on the doctors

The computer can help the doctors in their management of patients on long term repeat prescriptions, their supervision of at risk groups, and their planning for the future.

Repeat prescribing

The computer enables the practice to set up a system whereby patients only get onto repeat prescriptions as a positive decision, rather than drifting onto repeat prescriptions because their own doctor happens to be away at the time they run out.

Some patients may only come back for repeats at long intervals, for instance a man may have attacks of gout for which he needs a non-steroid anti-inflammatory. Such a patient may be started on his repeat prescription when his own doctor is on holiday, and even the most conscientious general practitioner using a manual system may never have seen him. Nor will he come to much harm. There are patients, however, who get on to repeat prescription drugs which do have side effects which should be monitored, often the drugs are being used inappropriately.

The computer can avoid this problem because the partners can agree that every patient on the repeat prescription register will have had their repeat prescription formally approved by their own doctor. There should be a built in facility for making sure the patients are seen at regular intervals.

There is an additional check on long term prescribing which is that the computer should be able to print out a list of all the drugs being used so that the doctor can look through them and confirm that nobody is on a drug he/she is unfamiliar with or one which he thinks should be monitored more closely. This facility is particularly useful if a drug is suddenly found to have serious side effects as the computer can do a rapid search to identify all patients who are currently on it.

Reviewing sets of patients with chronic disease

If the computer has facilities for making up a morbidity index the morbidity index can be made more accurate by doing searches. Thus checking for patients on repeat prescriptions for diabetic drugs will identify diabetics who have not yet got on to the morbidity index. This facility for cross checking is one of the computer's most powerful functions and if it is exploited fully it can greatly improve the care of those patients who would otherwise be lost to follow up.

The morbidity index itself can be used to set up a recall system for patients, for example diabetics, but in an average practice the numbers are so small that a manual system is probably easier.

Patients at special risk

An obvious group of patients at special risk are the elderly, nowadays defined as those over the age of 75. It is relatively easy using a computer to identify all the patients of a particular doctor who are over 75. They can then be divided into a subset of those already regularly reviewed, perhaps because they are on the morbidity index, and the remainder can be checked on either by the doctor him/herself or by the health visitor.

Planning for the future

Most doctors' lists of patients grow old with them, women doctors tend to have more women patients. Older patients generate more work. When a partner retires his list will move to a new young partner who should have the energy to cope with a more demanding older list perhaps with a preponderance of extremely old patients; meanwhile young families will come to him/her, especially if he or she is interested in obstetrics. This pattern of patient distribution has been an accepted part of general practice for years, but can easily get exaggerated so a particular partner can get overwhelmed, or at least feel overwhelmed, by one sort of patient. Typically a woman doctor gets many elderly women.

As a computerised system can very quickly generate an age–sex register the primary health care team can use it to plan for the future. Where there are differences in the structure of different partners' lists, it can be used so as to selectively direct patients towards a particular partner. This evens out the work load and makes the list easier to transfer to a new partner when somebody retires.

Effect on the whole health care team

Audit

Clearly having the age sex distribution of a list enables a primary health care team to predict the expected number of patients with specific diseases such as hypertension. This can then be compared with the actual numbers and give a measure of how well the practice is doing at case detection.

There are now programs that go one stage further by plotting a geographical distribution of the patients and comparing the expected numbers with the observed numbers in each area of the practice. In this way it has been shown that even in a town a natural barrier such as a hill may separate an area where many hypertensives have been identified, from one where only a few live. In this particular case it was thought that the number of patients from the area on the far side of the hill from the surgery seems to be less, because they come less often and so miss the opportunistic health screening they would otherwise have got. The same exercise with asthmatic children revealed that too few were being diagnosed in the poorer area of the town.

Future developments

Improving present systems

For the next few years much effort will be needed to improve the existing systems. It will be a long time before the present system of manual notes and their Lloyd George folders are replaced and the present computer systems in practice do not mix well with them. For example the summary sheet is usually printed on flimsy paper which gets lost in the notes. Another problem is remembering to transfer clinical data from the notes to the computer, this is a problem which will probably be overcome as soon as bar codes and their readers become cheap enough for every set of notes to be coded.

Exchange of data

At present there is no automatic exchange of data between Family Practitioner or local authority computers and general practitioner's computers. This means that data on inoculations have to be recorded twice. In the same way screening programmes such as cervical smear campaigns are inefficient because the present system involves letters being sent from Family Practitioner Committees to health centres when the test may already have been done.

Expert systems

After tremendous enthusiasm for programmes which would replace the doctor as diagnostician it seems that little progress has been made over the last 15 years. The work has thrown more light on how doctors make diagnoses but the main application of the research has been outside medicine, for example finding faults in telephone systems.[1]

Reference

1 Schwartz, W.B., Patil, R.S., Szolovits, P. Artificial Intelligence in Medicine. New England Journal of Medicine, 1987, **316**, 685–7.

CHAPTER 14

The Primary Health Care Team Now and In the Future

Changes in the traditional structure of the delivery of care

Primary health care teams are not the only organisations that are changing in the health service. Parallel changes are occurring in the specialist services so that the traditional arrangement of independent general practitioners referring to consultants is changing to one of a multi-disciplinary primary health care team referring patients to a multi-disciplinary secondary health care team.

The traditional system in its shortest form can be illustrated as in Figure 14.1. The general practitioner would see a patient, perhaps with a psychiatric problem. He would manage the patient himself if he could, but if not he would refer him or her to the psychiatrist. The psychiatrist could then be helped in his management of the case by ancillary workers; for example, he might have access to hospital beds and the inpatient staff, or to a clinical psychologist. These people would, however, be under his control and the general practitioner would not be able to make direct referrals to them.

The trend has now changed and the move in the secondary health tier is to work in teams of which the doctor is a member, but not always the leader (see Figure 14.2). Thus the psychiatrist will work in a team with psychologists, community psychiatric nurses, psychotherapists and occupational therapists. The paediatric team will consist of paediatricians, child psychologists, child dieticians and specialist social workers. The ear, nose and throat surgeon will work with the teacher for the deaf, and so on. Meanwhile members of the primary health care team are now able to refer direct to members of the secondary health care team instead of having to channel all referrals through the doctors.

Benefits and disadvantages of the change

The principal benefit of the change must be that it saves time, especially the patient's time. A patient with an injured shoulder who needs physiotherapy no longer has to wait to see an orthopaedic surgeon before again waiting for an appointment for treatment. Children with possible squints can be sent direct from a health visitor in her developmental clinic to the orthoptist.

The disadvantages are that certain services may be inappropriately overloaded. For example, the dietician may be asked to see so many obese people, for whom she can probably do very little, that she has no time for those with coeliac disease for whom she can do a great deal. If she had all her referrals from one person, a doctor, she could 'educate' that doctor. There is, however, little evidence that doctors are amenable to this sort of education, and anyway, where open access to facilities such as physiotherapy or X-ray services has been started, it has in most cases been properly used.

Figure 14.1   Traditional pattern

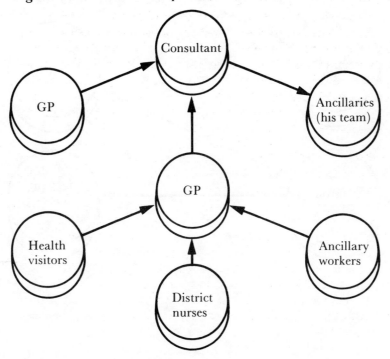

Figure 14.2   Evolving patterns and delivery of care

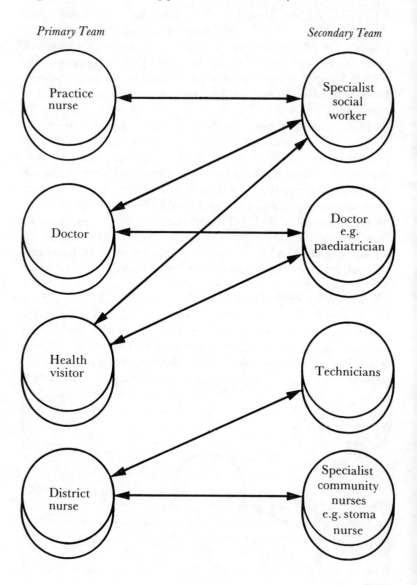

Transfer of the care of patients to the primary health care team and allocation of resources

Already 90% of all illness is dealt with in the community by the primary health care team. Admitting patients to hospital or even just sending them to outpatient departments costs a lot of money. If this money can be saved by discharging patients early, by not following them up, or by not even seeing them in hospital in the first place, there will be more money available for other services.

This is a powerful argument for doing as much as possible in the community and for expanding the role of the primary health care team. The members of the primary health care team will have to agree to accept much more responsibility and will sometimes need more training. They will also have more work, so teams will have to be larger with each person perhaps looking after fewer patients.

The objections to such a policy are that it may cost more to care for people in the community if more seriously ill patients are being looked after there. Specifically, if psychiatric patients are discharged they will often have to live in hostels which have to be bought, fitted out and staffed. Similarly, if chronically physically disabled are sent home they will need more district nursing support, more equipment and more home help. Money is not the only consideration. There is the question of safety. Do patients with uncomplicated myocardial infarctions do as well at home as in hospital? How safe are home confinements? The answers to both these questions depend largely on what is meant by uncomplicated and how easily complications can be predicted. There is also the question of quality of life. Although it is pleasanter to live at home with your family when you are chronically ill, or to have your baby in your own bed, at what point do you transfer resources and how far do you go? The Dutch system of having a large proportion of babies delivered at home is successful but expensive because it involves a comprehensive screening system, reliable transport to the hospital if there is a crisis, and paid maternity aids to help the midwife for at least eight hours a day for seven days after the delivery.

How effective is a primary health care team?

This question does not have clear cut answers, but it is important to know how to set about looking for answers. For example, we might do a double blind trial or look at equivalent outcomes or outcomes using external differences.

The double blind controlled trial

The ideal test of a new treatment is to submit it to a double blind controlled trial. In this the experimenter does not know into which treatment group the subject has been entered until the end of the experiment. This sort of experiment is difficult enough when new drugs are being tested; it would seem almost impossible in primary health care, especially as much of the illness seen is common and there are already established, indeed entrenched, systems of treatment. Nevertheless, there have been studies in the delivery of health care, in particular by the Rand Corporation in the USA who studied different systems of delivering primary health care. Broadly their findings were that the larger the patient's financial contribution at the time they used the service, the less use they made of it. Using the service less did not seem to affect their health. One interesting finding was that in pre-paid plans the higher-income sick people did better and the poor people did worse and were more likely to die.[1] The NHS is a pre-paid system, so this is an important finding. Do we really want a system that militates against the poor, for whom medicine has traditionally assumed a special responsibility?

Outcome of care

Another approach to the problem is to look at it in terms of outcome, to see whether a theoretical advantage of a system actually does what it is supposed to do. For example, British general practice is ideally structured for preventive medicine. General practitioners have a defined population on their list and there are several identifiable risk factors that they could easily look for, yet cardiovascular mortality has remained static in the UK but fallen in countries such as Australia and the USA where patients pay for every service that they get. This may have more to do with the personality of the people involved and it may be that British people are more resistant than others to health education programmes.

It is tempting to condemn all primary health care under the NHS on the basis of such studies. One particularly galling study in which non-insulin dependent diabetics were discharged randomly from a hospital clinic showed that those who remained under the care of secondary health care teams (the hospital diabetic clinic) had less illness and significantly lower mortality than those who were transferred to the care of their general practitioner.[2] However, another study published in the same edition of the *British Medical Journal* showed that where mini-clinics for diabetics were set up in the practices, control of the diabetes was just as good as in the hospital clinics.[3]

References

1 (1986) The Rand Health Insurance Study: A spanner in the works. *Lancet*, **i**; 1012 (Leading article).
2 Hayes, T.M. and Harries J. (1984) Randomised controlled trial of routine hospital clinic care versus routine general practice care for type II diabetics. *B. Med. J.*, **289**, 728–30.
3 Singh, B.M., Holland, M.R. and Thorn, P.A. (1984) Metabolic control of diabetes in general practice clinics: comparison with a hospital clinic. *B. Med. J.*, **289**; 726–8.

CHAPTER 15

The Receptionist

No job description can accurately set out what receptionists do. On the face of it their job is to give patients appointments and to get out the notes for the doctors, plus a few subsidiary tasks. In fact they are central to the running of the practice and much of their day is involved in negotiating between the very large number of people asking for the resources of the team and those providing it. Both the demand for services and their supply will fluctuate depending on the day of the week, who is on leave, and whether there is an epidemic on. The primary health care team will function better if its members understand some of the receptionists' problems.

What the job description says v. what receptionists actually do

The job description of the medical receptionist could read like this:

1. Make up appointments book by telephone or person to person for doctors and practice nurse.
2. Produce appointment lists and patients' notes for individual doctors.
3. Deal with repeat prescriptions.
4. General filing and numerous clerical duties.
5. Accept telephone calls on behalf of the health visitors and community nurses and enter details in calls book.
6. Oversee and supervise waiting area.

Although they will do and see all these things, much time and energy is also spent in dealing with chronic patients who can cope only by constant contact with the primary health care team. Some of these patients will just telephone in for a chat, others will call in, while yet others will go to further lengths and

Figure 15.1 The wasteful 'Y' situation

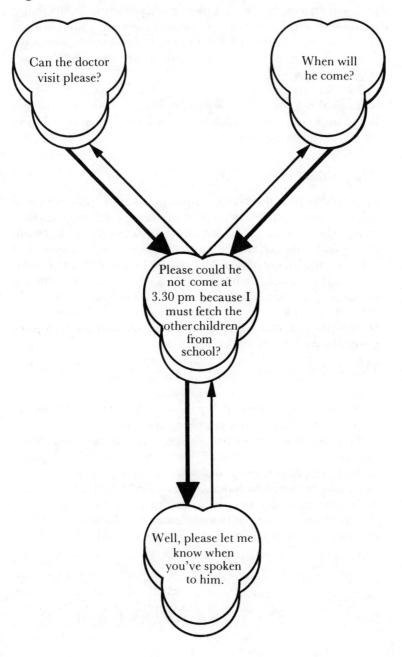

devise elaborate strategies for keeping on ringing up. Perhaps they will arrange for their regular repeat prescription medicines to run out at different times, or produce new symptoms or even just come in to check on the time of their next appointment. Many of these essentially lonely people are effectively carried by a good reception staff.

The receptionist will also have to exercise much diplomacy when dealing with the people on her side of the counter, toning down unreasonable sounding requests and generally offering encouragement.

Theoretical considerations

It has been shown that where people sit in a circle and feed information to each other problems are solved more quickly than if they sit in a 'Y' arrangement feeding information to an individual who collates it and sends it back to them. The receptionists are often in a 'Y' situation. Patients ring to ask to speak with a doctor or health visitor. The receptionist buzzes the doctor on the internal line and asks if he can take the call. He is in the middle of a consultation and asks the patient to ring back at a particular time, or alternatively, suggests he or she make an appointment to see him. The receptionist then negotiates a suitable appointment with the patient. This is a simplified example, but it is what happens all day long.

Demands also come from the primary health care workers: 'Try to keep my surgery short today please.' 'Can you get the doctor to do some more developmentals?' 'Please make sure the district nurse gets this message soon, and let me know if she cannot get there this morning.' The receptionist has to balance these competing or even incompatible demands against each other and negotiate with the various people involved. All this is time consuming and usually inefficient.

There are ways in which things can be improved and an obvious one is to channel as little as possible through the receptionists. The second way is to lay down broad policies and stick to them. For example, it might be decided that the doctor would not receive telephone calls while consulting unless the receptionist had first asked the patient if she could take a message, or ask if the doctor can ring back. In another practice the doctors may agree to accept all telephone calls in the hope that it might save their time in the long run.

Laying down policies can give rise to a further problem, which is that the more protocols that are set up, the more problems the receptionists will have in remembering them. The doctors have to have the same policy or none at all.

The receptionist's most effective strategy from her own point of view is probably to direct people to by-pass her as much as possible. For example, if patients wish to know whether they should see the health visitor the call can be put through directly to him or her. This means that the receptionists have to abnegate not only some of their power but also some of their expertise as one of their main functions is to solve problems for others and to answer questions. Furthermore, if people by-pass the receptionist she will miss out on some information.

Responsibility and authority

The more the receptionist knows the more responsibility she can take on. Sometimes she will be asked for information by patients, information such as whether there is an influenza epidemic or whether something is poisonous. As she is the first point of contact in the primary health care team her answers will carry authority, even though the people she is speaking to may realise that she is as much a lay person as they are. It is often very difficult to know whether there is an epidemic going on and whether a particular substance is poisonous. The receptionist may be well aware of this and not wish to mislead, but she will also want to be helpful.

One thing she always does is to control information, specifically on the availability or whereabouts of the doctors. In a well run primary health team all members of staff are reasonably accessible and it is always possible for a patient to see his or her own doctor or health visitor within 24 hours. In an emergency a doctor, not necessarily the patient's own, would be available much sooner. If the doctors for various reasons decide not to be so readily accessible, more responsibility is put onto the receptionists who may eventually be making major decisions about what is urgent and what is trivial.

Although the doctors' and the patients' wishes do coincide in that both want the patient to be as healthy as possible and to come for treatment as rarely as possible, their interests can clash: whereas the doctors will wish to conserve their energy and will be asking the receptionists not to overload them, the patients will feel that they are competing for a resource and that they also have no information about how available it is.

How the receptionists are paid

Receptionists are appointed and paid by the medical practitioners, although the practice manager will do most of the work of advertising, short listing and interviewing. There are no fixed rules about how much a receptionist should be paid, and the partnership can claim back up to 70% from the Family Practitioner Committee. Usually the receptionist will be employed on the Whitley Council Scale grades, and some Family Practitioner Committees are allowing the claims only if the salary is within that Scale. These scales apply to public employees in the NHS and are re-negotiated regularly. This means that there is an outside body which controls rises in salary and it makes the relationship in the practice that much easier. Although General Practitioners can claim back 70% of what they pay their ancillary staff, they are limited to employing people on this basis to 74 hours per week per doctor.

Who the receptionists are responsible to

The chain of responsibility will vary in different practices but usually the receptionists will be responsible to the senior receptionist who will be paid more and who will have the job of organising the reception area and the day to day work. She in her turn will be responsible to the practice manager. It is useful to have a statement in all the job descriptions stating the chain of command, and also making the point that if there is a dispute the receptionists do have a right to put the problem directly to a partner who should then bring it to the next partners' meeting. The receptionist is in one of the few hierarchical structures in the primary health care team.

Training and career structure for receptionists

At present there are no full time training courses for receptionists. In several parts of the country there are half-day release courses for receptionists who are already in post. These extend over a period of up to 18 months and the topics covered include such things as medical terminology, the structure and organisation of the health service and different ways of running a practice.

The doctors are re-imbursed in part for the receptionists' salaries, but they are not re-imbursed for such things as pensions. Some receptionists will be unmarried or newly married and will expect to stay for only a few years until they start having children. The majority, however, will be older women, often with grown children, who may be there until retirement. After a few years their annual increments in salary will stop and, after becoming a senior receptionist, they will have no further promotion except to become a practice manager. Although in the past many senior receptionists became practice managers, the skills are different; the practice manager has less contact with the public and needs more in the way of accounting and administrative skills.

There is much to be said for having several part-time receptionists. This suits many women who still have children at home and who have husbands in demanding jobs. Working as a receptionist is emotionally demanding and part-timers do shorter shifts. More people are available for holiday relief and to do extra hours if somebody is sick.

Against having larger numbers of receptionists are the problems of communication. This applies not only to practice policies, which will be more difficult to promulgate, but also day-to-day information about problems with patients.

Reference

1 Sidney, E., Brown, M. and Argyle, M. (1979) *Skills with people—a guide for managers*. London, Hutchinson, pp 129.

CHAPTER 16

The Practice Nurse

The practice nurse was almost unknown until the mid-1970s, when it began to be realised that a fully trained nurse could be employed by the general practitioner and 70% of her pay be reimbursed. In some countries, particularly the USA, doctors employ nurses to act as personal assistants: they work with the doctor in a subsidiary role bringing in patients from the waiting room and doing simple preliminary examinations such as weighing and taking blood pressures and temperatures. The modern British practice nurse does no reception work; she is more an independent practitioner in her own right. She may work in a room in premises owned by the doctors and be paid by them, but she is most effective in her role as another person to whom patients have direct access.

Treatment as against diagnosis

The professional role of the nurse is to treat patients and care for them rather than to make diagnoses. The practice nurse will spend most of her time giving or supervising treatment, but in many cases she will also be asked for advice and make diagnostic decisions. The range of conditions she may be consulted about may be wide and include such problems as rashes, boils, deafness and vaginal discharges. Many of these are within her competence; for example, she may become more skilled than the doctor at taking vaginal swabs and deciding whether patients' breasts are normal. With more women doctors in general practice it is easier for women patients to see a doctor about gynaecological and other problems that they would be unwilling to take to a man. Nevertheless, there is still a large unfulfilled demand for advice on women's problems. A practice nurse helps fill this gap.

One major advantage for the nurse of working in the same

building as the doctors is that she can ask the doctors immediately if there is a problem and perhaps persuade the patient to see one of them.

She will sometimes be asked about conditions that patients feel are too trivial to bother the doctors with. This can lead to problems. Firstly, the nurse is usually busier than the doctors and, secondly, what appears trivial to the patient may be the first symptom of serious disease, for example a change in bowel habit or the passing of blood. Thus allowing patients direct access to the nurse could go badly wrong if the nurse is not properly trained or allows herself to get rushed.

Payment of the practice nurse

Practice nurses are employed by the doctors and therefore responsible to them. The doctors reclaim 70% of the nurses' pay from the Family Practitioner Committee. The nurses are usually paid at ward sister level on the Whitley Council Scale.

The advantages of this system are that the practice nurse knows the people she is responsible to (if she was paid from, say, the Area Health Authority, she would be dealing with a relatively unknown official) and, as the doctors have to contribute to her pay, they are more likely to check that they and their patients are getting value for money. Against these advantages must be set the anomaly that often the nurse is doing things such as giving injections or doing cervical smears for which the doctors then claim an item-of-service fee.

Training the practice nurse

As the practice nurse is a relatively new phenomenon there is as yet no formal training. Although the practical skills of the practice nurse are relatively clear cut, the extent of her role as a diagnostician and counsellor are still blurred. It is relatively easy for the general practitioner she is working with to help her learn how to do venepunctures or take cervical smears, but he or she can have little idea about the broader aspects of her job.

The solution to this problem is for practice nurses to define their own role and devise their own training schemes. This is already being done through local practice nurse groups. The contents of the syllabus will obviously change with time, but the main modules are as follows:

Attitudes

The practice nurse has to be able to work as an independent practitioner. She has to have the administrative ability and attitude to run her own department. She has to organise and stock the treatment room, make sure that she has an effective appointments system and that an adequate service is provided for the patients. This usually involves liaising with other nurses so that proper cover is provided. She has to make sure that her skills are fully utilised and yet be aware of her limitations. She has to make sure her knowledge keeps up to date and that she is not doing procedures she is not properly trained for.

Skills

The practice nurse has to know how to do such things as:

Take and record blood pressure
Weigh patients and give dietary advice
Venepuncture
Urine tests and take mid-stream urine specimens
Vaginal examinations and take high vaginal swabs
Cervical smear tests
Instruct in self-examination of breasts
ECG
Allergy testing
Ear syringing
Evert eyelid and irrigate eye
Remove sutures
Injections—intradermal, subcutaneous and intramuscular
Immunisations—routine tetanus and travellers abroad
Dressings—leg ulcers, burns, boils and abscesses
Treat warts
Assist doctors in minor operations, fit IUDs and do post-
    natal examinations
Family planning—information, advice, fit and teach about
    caps
Change vaginal ring pessaries

Knowledge

The practice nurse has to have the background knowledge to support new skills. For example, she should be aware of changes in requirements for travellers' immunisation and in new developments in contraceptive technique or the management of hypertension.

Much of the training of practice nurses by one another takes place in their own time. The practice that employs them can claim 70% reimbursement of travelling expenses and subsistence. As the need for training becomes more obvious it is likely that more courses will be arranged during the working day so that training and peer review can be formally recognised as an important part of the job.

CHAPTER 17

The Health Visitor

The striking features of the modern health visitor are her informal approach and the breadth of her task.

Health visitors used to wear uniforms, perhaps a legacy of their nursing background, but nowadays nursing uniforms are thought to put people off and the tendency is to dress like everybody else. Perhaps because of their informality, the range of jobs given to them has increased enormously.

Training

The basic qualification to become a health visitor is a nursing training to Registered General Nurse standard. She also needs experience in midwifery. She then has to have some practical nursing experience before going on to do a one year polytechnic or university course. In most instances she will be sponsored by a health authority.

Tasks that are the responsibility of the health visitor

Although health visitors regard themselves as able and willing to advise and support all age groups from preconception to extreme old age, much of their work is with the most vulnerable groups in society—small children, their mothers, and the very old and frail. Learning how to look after children is best begun before they are even born and this is why health visitors go one stage further and run parentcraft sessions for pregnant women and their partners on an informal programmed basis. These are organised in cooperation with the midwife.

Once the baby has been born there is a statutory requirement for the midwife to visit every day including the

10th day. This policy varies in different health authorities and midwives may visit until the 28th day. On the 11th day the health visitor will make her first call and from then on will provide advice and support until the child goes to school.

Other vulnerable groups the health visitor comes into contact with and provides extra support for are the unemployed, single parents and the socially deprived.

Developmental screening of the under 5s

Developmental screening is a team activity for which the health visitors have the main responsibility but in which the doctors are also involved. Typically, children are seen at:

Six weeks	Mainly for physical examination to identify congenital abnormalities. Specifically examination of the hips and heart.
Seven months	First routine hearing check (distraction test) and a review of development, also observing for squints.
One year or 18 months	Developmental birthday check looking for squints etc.
Three years	Developmental birthday check including routine test of vision, hearing and behaviour.
Four years	Pre-school check involving complete examination by the doctor and a report being sent to the local teacher warning him/her about possible problems such as speech difficulties. (Sheridan or Denver screening is used by most health visitors.)

Other people do screening tests on the children (examination by the doctor at birth, and a PKU (phenylketonuria) and hypothyroid test at eight days by the midwife), but the main burden falls on the health visitor.

When the child goes to school the health visitor hands care over to the school nurse, who will check visual acuity yearly and colour vision at eight years, while an audiology technician will test hearing at six years. Health visitors keep in touch with the schools as part of their liaison network. This is particularly valuable where problems occur in families as the health visitor can act as a line of communication from the primary health care team to the teacher.

Postnatals, parentcraft, feeding problems and emotional development

Often, until a woman has actually had a baby, she does not understand what the problems are. For many women mothering does not come naturally and even nurses and women doctors who have had a lot of information can have problems. One of the most valuable functions of the 11th day visit is that it introduces the mother to the idea that expert help is available. Some of her problems can be brought to the weekly well baby clinics where babies are weighed and growth is monitored.

The well baby clinic has another use which is to give mothers of toddlers a chance to meet each other. Much has been written about the dramatic change in lifestyle that occurs when a woman becomes a housewife and a mother.[1] There is mainly a feeling of vulnerability and loss of status. Postnatal groups can help to reduce this feeling and this is important because if the mother can feel happy and secure in her role she will rear a happy and secure person in her baby. Society has learnt the lesson of giving privileges to women antenatally, but has not yet begun to give privileges in the postnatal phase.

Immunisation and follow-up of defaulters

A good primary health care team can achieve levels of immunisation approaching 97%. This depends on good organisation and often on using a computer. It also depends on good education by the health visitors. Many parents will be worried about the risks involved in immunisation and will have heard less of the benefits than of the complications. Some children will be unsuitable for immunisation, for instance any child who has had a fit or who has a family history of epilepsy should not have pertussis vaccination. The health visitor is responsible for identifying children who have not arrived for immunisation and following them up by visiting them at home. This is a part of the job that some health visitors do not like, perhaps because it carries an image of police work.

Meetings and liaison

As health visitors are involved across such a wide field they are involved in numerous meetings with each other and various specialist agencies. They may have liaison meetings in the paediatric, maternity and geriatric departments at the district general hospital. There will also be liaison meetings with those running playgroups and with health visitors attached to schools. A thriving health visitor group will also have weekly meetings and perhaps a monthly journal club.

The elderly

Much emphasis has been placed on prevention in the elderly, but it seems that screening does not find much pre-symptomatic illness. On the other hand, many elderly people decline slowly, and if the health visitors visit them they can anticipate problems and avoid crises. For example, in a cold snap the client may suddenly be unable to cope. The result is an old person going into an overcrowded hospital, perhaps in a state of hypothermia. It saves money and upset if old people can go on living in their own homes as long as possible, but there comes a time when they start depending on the goodwill of their neighbours, many of whom may be almost as old as they are. Health visitors are able to assess the situation and sometimes make simple suggestions that help old people keep their independence longer, such as installing storage heaters in place of solid fuel heating or using home help or meals on wheels. They are also in a position to broach the subject of moving to a warden-supervised flat or even into a nursing home. Health visitors are experts in that vague area between medicine and social work.

How health visitors are paid and who they are responsible to

Health visitors are paid by their area health authority. They have their own salary grading on a similar level to ward sister I–II, which is something of an anomaly as their training is longer and they have more clients.

Their contracts are held at area level and they are

responsible to the local nursing management team. In practice, however, there is usually little interference in their day-to-day work and much freedom to work using their own initiative in the best interests of the clients or patients. A good working relationship with the general practitioner, the district nursing sister, the practice nurse and all the primary health care team is essential and inspires everyone to give the best possible service to the patient.

Reference

1 Oakley, A. (1974) *Housewife*. London, Allen Lane.

Further Reading

Colver, A.F. and Steiner, H. (1986) Health surveillance of preschool children. *Br. Med. J.* **293**; 258–60.

CHAPTER 18

The Community Psychiatric Nurse

Although community psychiatric nurses are vital members of the primary health care team they are in an anomalous position because they are usually employed and paid by a hospital. They are thus members of a secondary health care team. From the hospital's point of view they are there to keep people out of hospital beds but they can do this effectively only by working in close contact with the primary team and by practising anticipatory care as against preventive care. This is a relatively recent change and is partly due to their having learnt skills such as how to do family therapy or to run groups that would be wasted if they spent their time as follow-up nurses.

Recruitment and training

Community psychiatric nurses are all registered mental nurses who have expressed an interest in working in the community. They usually undergo a one year course in training, often based in a polytechnic. The course usually comprises an academic component and a series of placements in various departments such as the social services. The academic component includes sociology and psychology as well as some project work.

Although community psychiatric nurses will see their job mainly in terms of nursing assessment, treatment and monitoring of psychiatric patients in the community, many of them will acquire more specialist skills in areas such as family therapy and counselling. One of the reasons that psychiatric nurses are attracted to community psychiatric nursing is because it gives them independence and flexibility. Working with in-patients is different in that the patients tend to be more seriously ill and their treatment involves the use of drugs more than group work and psychotherapy.

Payment

At present community psychiatric nurses are usually paid from the hospital budget. This means that they are responsible to a clinical nurse manager with responsibility for the community.

How the community psychiatric nurse spends the day

Unlike other health care workers the community psychiatric nurse has a relatively unstructured day (see Figure 18.1). There are regular slots for meetings and also for formal therapy sessions, but much of the time has to be kept available for crisis intervention, either in the hospital or in the community. Clearly the main part of visiting will involve patients who have been under treatment during the acute phase of their illness and who are now back at home living either alone or with their families. Some of these patients will be schizophrenic or severely depressed and, although the community psychiatric nurse will be seeing them and checking on their treatment, he or she will also expect to spend time and effort discussing the problems with relatives who may easily need more support and advice than the patients themselves. The other category of patient who needs to be seen at home is the patient who is very nearly unable to care for him/herself because of progressive dementia. Many elderly patients can just cope with life in the community but become at risk if there is even a minor change in their circumstances, such as a spell of unusual weather. They may then need to go back into hospital at short notice. The advantage of the community psychiatric nurse seeing them regularly is that they are able to negotiate such re-admissions without too much difficulty.

Formal therapy

Community psychiatric nurses do different types of formal therapy depending on their training and inclination. Group work, which obviously requires experience and training, may appeal to one whereas another may wish to acquire skills in family therapy. Even when working with families each community psychiatric nurse may work more comfortably with

Figure 18.1 How the community psychiatric nurse spends her day

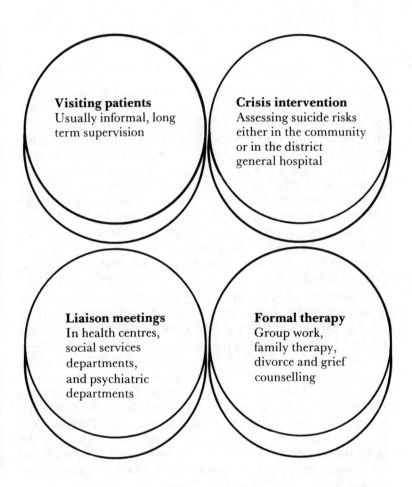

Visiting patients
Usually informal, long term supervision

Crisis intervention
Assessing suicide risks either in the community or in the district general hospital

Liaison meetings
In health centres, social services departments, and psychiatric departments

Formal therapy
Group work, family therapy, divorce and grief counselling

one technique than with another. One may use modern technology—for example, interviewing families in rooms with one-way mirrors so that his or her efforts can be supervised and even modified during the interview by hidden observers. Another may prefer to work by getting him/herself involved in the emotional tangles of the family and then using this to help the family identify what they do to each other.

CHAPTER 19

The General Practitioner

Although there are now 29 000 general practitioners working in the UK, there is surprisingly little information about how they work, the hours they put in and the amount they do for their patients.

There are big differences in the number of patients they care for and the amount of time they give to each patient in a year, or indeed at a consultation. Broadly, the longer the doctor's list the less time given to each patient, but this pattern is not consistent and it seems that there are doctors with small lists who spend little time even with those patients they do see. Other doctors with lists of above average size and with outside commitments, for instance hospital work, have longer appointments for their patients and seem to do more.

This says nothing about how good the care is, although it seems obvious that when appointments get below a certain duration more of each one will be spent greeting the patient and saying goodbye than on medical matters.

Such work as has been done on the quality of care in general practice shows that doctors vary widely in their abilities. Very few doctors, for example, correctly identify all the psychiatric patients who consult them and those who identify more patients as having psychiatric illness do not always do so correctly, sometimes missing cases and sometimes making the wrong diagnosis.[1]

General practitioner trainees

In 1981 the Vocational Training Act made it compulsory for all doctors entering general practice to have completed a recognised three-year course of training. The training had to consist of two years in approved hospital posts and one year in a training practice. Responsibility for approving both the hospital and the general practice posts was delegated to regional committees who laid down their own criteria.

It is estimated that about one practice in four is a training practice. This is about the right ratio to train enough young doctors to replace retiring principals.

The practice has to meet nationally agreed and regional criteria. At present the national criteria refer only to the standard of notes, which have to be fixed in chronological order and, in due course, include an attached summary of diseases that the patient has had. The regional criteria vary and can extend to a whole handbook setting out minimum standards and suggested standards to aim at. They relate, firstly, to the ability of the trainer to teach, and his commitment; secondly, to the practice as a suitable learning environment; and, thirdly, to the standards of the practice as a primary health care team. The trainer is expected to devote an average of two-and-a-half hours a week to teaching the trainee by giving tutorials, doing joint surgeries and visits or, for example, reviewing cases. The trainee is employed by his trainer, who receives full reimbursement of his salary from the Family Practitioner Committee. The trainer is also paid to do the training.

It seems that the trainer is a very important, perhaps the most important, influence on the trainee and his/her future pattern of practice. As, despite many years of training in hospitals and medical school, it takes only a few months in a training practice for the trainee's patterns of prescribing antibiotics to match those of his trainer (personal comunication, M. Whitfield), attitudes to patients, consulting and notes probably follow the same pattern. Changing primary health care in the future therefore depends on changing the attitudes and methods of trainers now.

The general practitioner

The general practitioner in the UK is self-employed. After completing his training he can usually find employment only by replacing a retiring partner. There are still a very few areas in the country where a doctor can apply to the local family practitioner committee and set up on his own. In most of the country there are restrictions so that even if a doctor retires from a practice, his partners have to apply for a replacement.

The general practitioner's work can be divided into two broad categories. On the one hand there are the broadly based managerial responsibilities of cooperation with the rest of the team in the care of the patients on his list, especially those who do not come to the surgery. On the other hand there is the day-to-day management of patients who present at the medical centre or who are known to be ill. Central to this second task is the consultation.

The consultation

There is considerable variation in the number of patients doctors see per hour. Some docotrs see 12 or more and others less than six. Byrne and Long did a classic study on consultations[1] and were able to divide them into those that were functional—that is to say, both the doctor and the patient thought they had been effective and satisfying—and dysfunctional, where the doctor and the patient felt that the opposite had occurred. The most striking finding of their study was that a doctor who had many functional consultations did not always spend a long time with every patient and his consultations varied enormously in length. This commonsense finding is often ignored by general practitioners, who somehow seem to think that all encounters with patients have to be fitted into a rigid time framework.

Other studies have shown big variations in the amount of responsibility general practitioners are willing to take for the long term management of their patients, or indeed the short term care. Some doctors refer one patient in four to the outpatients department for a further opinion and treatment, others as few as one in 50.[2]

One of the most interesting findings about the way doctors behave in consultations is that they tend to retain the same pattern of behaviour no matter whom they are seeing, and that doctors are quite extraordinarily variable in the emphasis they put on different aspects of their task. In their book *The Consultation*,[3] which is well worth reading, a group of GPs describes how, by using video tapes of consultations, they were able, firstly, to show that these differences exist and, secondly, to identify a full list of the tasks of the consultation. These tasks are: identifying the patient's concerns and expectations; looking at ongoing problems; and looking at the patient's ideas of what is going on and involving him or her in the management of his or her own problem. The full list appears in the book,[3] but Figure 19.1 makes the point that different doctors emphasise different aspects of their contact with the patient. Thus one doctor will spend a lot of time looking at the disease and its cause without considering what the patient feels about it. He may prescribe without making sure that the patient understands and agrees with what is to happen. Such a doctor will probably have a low level of compliance with his treatment. The doctor represented in the diagram may spend much time identifying the patient's concerns but ignore ongoing problems such as his or her obesity or diabetes. He will fall into a different trap.

The general practitioner as a manager

The traditional role of the general practitioner in the British primary health care team is one of control and direction. The emphasis now is for the general practitioner to relinquish some of that control and to share decision making with other members of the team. One of the problems is that the general practitioner's income is determined by the profits of the practice and this is dependent on the way some of the members of the team direct their time and energy. This is particularly true for activities for which there are items-of-service payments. The general practioner will therefore want to keep some control over these team members.

Keeping control does not rule out *delegation*, and an important managerial skill for the general practitioner is learning to delegate. Doctors do not like delegation because they often feel they know more about a particular job than the people they plan to delegate it to. This is true at first but often, if the task is something that can be *clearly described* and the person who is taking it over is *able to learn the skills* from doing it, he or she may quite quickly become better at it than the doctor. It is also essential that the person to whom the task is delegated is

Figure 19.1   Differing emphasis on the tasks of the consultation

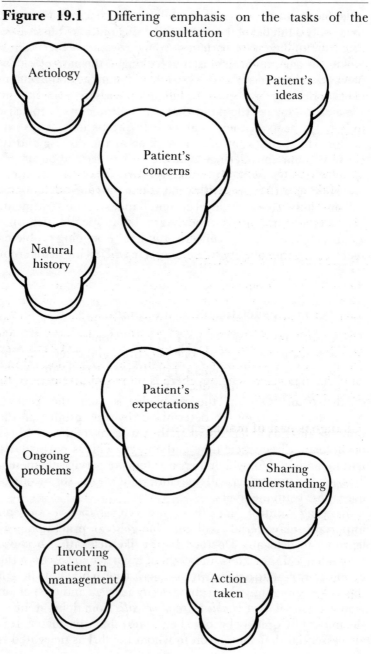

given the tools to do it properly. Thus a practice manager has to be given the authority and backing that he or she needs to direct the staff under him or her. Equally the practice nurse has to be given not just equipment and a room, but also time to go on courses to learn skills such as family planning or doing cervical smears. She too will need backing and authority to set up her clinics her way.

Guidelines for delegation

1. Decide what is to be delegated.
2. Describe the job and identify the skills needed to do it.
3. Make sure that the person who takes it on can and does learn how to do it.
4. Leave them to get on with it.

Repayment for ancillary workers

General Practitioners can claim back 70% of what they pay their ancillary staff, but they are limited to only employing people for seventy-four hours per week. Up until now there has been no query about employing reception staff, secretaries and practice nurses, but some Family Practitioner Committees have refused to re-imburse people such as Counsellors. Where staff have pension schemes there is no re-imbursement of the cost of the scheme.

Change is part of management

Management is a process of continuous adjustment. People change and attitudes change. Problems are looked at in different ways and new solutions appear. This means that part of the role of the team members, and particularly the doctors, is to look all the time at possibilities for improvement. This is a difficult lesson for general practitioners, whose training is often based on the idea that there is only one way to do things well and once that way has been identified it can be adopted forever.

Good management teams are changing their methods and ideas all the time.

References

1 Byrne, P.S. and Long, B.E.L. (1976) *Doctors talking to patients.* London, H.M.S.O.
2 Acheson, D. (1985) Variations in hospital referrals. In Teeling-Smith, G.Ed. *Health Education and general practice.* London, Office of Health Economics.
3 Pendleton D., Schofield T., Tate, P., and Hovelocks P. (1984) *The consultation; an approach to learning and teaching.* Oxford, Oxford University Press.

CHAPTER 20

Marriage Guidance

Even though the Marriage Guidance Council is a voluntary organisation, there is no doubt that it is complementary to the primary health care team. From time to time there have been moves to incorporate marriage guidance into the health service and some practices have and do employ counsellors.

Breakdown in a marriage is relatively common as marriage is probably the most demanding of all personal relationships. The consequences of such a breakdown on the health of the victims are far reaching, especially for children.[1] Apart from everything else there is often a dramatic fall in income, so that the standard of living of all involved declines and many expectations have to go unfulfilled.

The primary health care team, especially the health visitors and doctors, often get hints of impending trouble long before there is an actual breakdown: depression, difficulty in sleeping, sudden problems with contraception, sometimes even actual physical violence. It is worth remembering that even if a marriage gets to the stage where a woman is being hit by her husband it is still potentially viable. Indeed, in some ways the more intense a couple's feelings are towards each other the more hopeful the situation; it is only when one partner is indifferent to the other that little can be done.

Underlying philosophy

To the observer a marriage is a contract between two consenting adults. In reality people bring to their marriage many preconceptions and expectations. They get these ideas of marriage from different sources but clearly the most important is from their own homes and childhood experiences. Thus a woman will have a model of how a man should behave derived mainly from how her father behaved, but also from what she has seen on television and from other people. She may also feel that there are certain deficiencies in her father, perhaps he was never at home or tended to ignore her unless she made life a bit difficult for him, perhaps by a bit of extravagant spending.

The man in the marriage will also bring his own experiences of his mother, but perhaps in his case he may, for example, feel that his mother was not as demonstrative as he would have liked.

In most cases the split between expectations and reality is acceptable and two-thirds of marriages survive well. Inevitably, however, there are marriages where, though at first things go well, the signals the couple give each other become mixed up as soon as there are outside stresses, such as having children. The couple may, for instance, get much satisfaction at first because they are able to give each other a lot of time and attention which they both lacked as children. At a time of crisis such as when the wife becomes pregnant she may become less demonstrative and the husband will respond in the way he did to his own mother, perhaps by staying out late or by sulking. This could precipitate the wife into a bout of extravagance, and so on.

Thus the successful marriage has to fulfil the partners' needs at several levels. The more urgent the needs the more vulnerable the marriage.

The aim of marriage guidance counselling is to help people identify their needs and expectations so that they can see if there are more realistic ways of satisfying those needs and so that they can modify their expectations. It is the unconscious conflicts that the marriage guidance counsellor will look at.

Case history

John and Sara had been married for seven years. The marriage had appeared comfortable and successful. Sara presented at the doctor's surgery with bruises over her chest and breasts where John had beaten her. After a further similar episode they accepted that they needed help and went for marriage guidance. It took nine sessions to sort things out.

Going back to John's childhood, his mother had died of breast cancer when he was 11 years old, shortly after which he had failed to get into a grammar school. He was the second son and had been sent to live with relatives; he had been made to feel that he was only with them on sufferance and had not been able to express his feelings of anger and depression at his loss.

He had then taken on an apprenticeship and become a skilled craftsman, popular and successful at work. It was when he lost his job because of redundancy that the trouble with Sara began. She had come from a home where women were somewhat subservient and had looked to him for strength and capability. The marital fit had been good because his job had given him confidence and optimism, which he had needed to sustain his own image. It was the loss of his job that relit the anger and depression which he had never been able to express.

Once John recognised his desperate unmet need and Sara realised how her complementary problems and dependency had made things worse they were able to start reconstructing their relationship.

What is needed of the clients?

Nothing can be achieved if the client is not willing to put in a lot of work. He or she really has to want to make a go of it. Clients are probably going to be made very uncomfortable because they will have to start looking at themselves and realising that in some ways they may have been behaving like babies. In other ways they may have had great difficulty in behaving like babies and may have survived only because they had cut that part of their personality off from the rest of themselves. Losing some of these restraints may be even more difficult.

What is needed of the marriage guidance counsellor?

Marriage guidance counsellors are unpaid volunteers. They are expected to put in at least three sessions a week. They undergo an extended in-service training, but first go through a selection process usually involving several interviews and a day-long selection conference.

Counselling is time consuming and the training involves considerable emotional discomfort for the potential counsellor who has to go through the same process as the clients in order to get insight into how he or she behaves and why. If the client has to be strongly motivated it is perhaps appropriate to look at the motivation of the counsellor. This is something they have to do for themselves. Much of the work is initially interesting, as is all

Table 20.1 The categories of sexual dysfunction that are amenable to treatment

Men	Women
Impotence, primary	Vaginismus
secondary	
Premature ejaculation	Dyspareunia
Retarded ejaculation	Orgasmic difficulties
Inhibited desire	Inhibited desire

contact with other people, but it is likely that many counsellors become interested because they themselves have unresolved emotional conflicts, as do other primary health care workers.

Sexual problems

It has been said that quarrels in marriage revolve around three issues: money, sex, or alcohol abuse. Whether or not this is true, there is widespread ignorance about sexual function, in some ways made worse by the present climate of more frequent discussion of birth control techniques and the emphasis on sexual achievement in modern films and books. It has resulted in a generation that dares not admit ignorance about sex and sexuality.

At the same time there has been an increased tolerance of homosexuality and higher expectations of sexual satisfaction by women. On balance people are probably happier now in their sex lives than they used to be, but there are still many who can be helped.

The Marriage Guidance Council and the Family Planning Association were both quick to start using the techniques of Masters and Johnson when they first published their findings in the early 70s. Since then both organisations have gained much experience, and they have found it necessary to allocate workers entirely to sexual counselling, and to marital sexual therapy which uses a behavioural approach rather than the client-centred psychodynamic approach of counselling.

Obviously there are often emotional problems related to the physical problems and sometimes sexual problems are due to difficulties both the partners have in just telling each other what they want and need. On the other hand there are some sexual problems that are due to ignorance or just unsatisfactory first experiences. These are often readily treated (and usually overcome provided there is no pathology in the marriage) after only a few sessions. Top of the list of such problems is premature ejaculation by the man.

What happens when a marriage guidance counsellor is seen

There is often a waiting list for a few weeks for an appointment to see a counsellor. Generally speaking it is better for the clients to make the appointment themselves as they will need to take responsibility for their own destiny and making the first appointment is a good start.

A referral letter from the general practitioner to the counsellor can indicate the degree of urgency in the case and is therefore appreciated. It also tells the counsellor it was the general practitioner who referred the case. The letter need not be comprehensive; in fact it is probably better if it is brief and has few details.

Counsellors work in different ways but a common pattern is for the first meeting to be used to identify the problem and the clients' expectations.

The initial interview of half an hour is usually by a more experienced counsellor. This diagnostic interview may then result in the patient being accepted for therapy or referred elsewhere. Some patients are not suitable for marriage guidance, for example, if they do not wish to make a go of their relationship and need to see a lawyer, or if they are already seeing a psychotherapist.

If the marriage appears to have no pathology but there are sex problems they will be referred to a sexual therapist; otherwise they will be given an appointment to see a counsellor. There will be about six to eight subsequent sessions, each for one hour.

Counsellors are not paid and the Marriage Guidance Association is supported by voluntary contributions. Clients are expected to make a contribution towards the cost of each interview, although this is negotaible depending on their income and can be waived if there is a real financial problem.

Popular misconceptions

Some people are reluctant to go for marriage guidance because they believe that the counsellor will see them only as a couple rather than individually. This is not the case, as it is very common for one partner to go on his or her own.

Other reasons given for not going to marriage guidance are that the situation is not bad enough or, alternatively, that it has gone too far already.

Marriage guidance counsellors are willing to see, and indeed frequently do see, clients who are undergoing divorce and want help from a counsellor to understand why their marriage has ended.

Reference

1 Caplan, G. (1986) Preventing psychological problems in children of divorce: the general practioner's role. *Br. Med. J.*, **292**; 1431–4; 1563–6.

Further Reading

Skynner, R. (1976) *One flesh, separate persons*. London, Constable.
Skynner, R., and Cleese, J. (1983) *Families and how to survive them*. London, Methuen.

The second of these books is written in a more colloquial style, which is intended to make it easier to read. The Marriage Guidance Council supplies literature and introductory handouts.

CHAPTER 21

The District Nurse

Without district nurses it would be impossible for some patients to be cared for in their homes. The costs of looking after patients in hospital are now so high that every effort is made to keep them at home and to send them home early after treatment, especially after surgery. This would be impossible without the district nursing service. The increased work has not been matched by an increase in the numbers of district nurses. Most district nurses are women, which is why the feminine gender will be used in this chapter, but as more men enter the profession so more of them become district nurses. Male district nurses are particularly valuable in dealing with elderly incontinent men who need catheterisation. It is difficult for them to look after women because of the problems of embarrassment and the need for chaperones.

How the district nurse spends her day

The most important attribute of an effective district nurse must be the ability to be flexible. At one extreme some patients have to be seen at specific times of the day, particularly diabetics to whom she gives insulin. These patients are often elderly and blind. They cannot cope with changes in routine. At the other extreme the district nurse will be asked to see an acutely ill patient, perhaps somebody who has had a stroke, whose family need immediate help. The district nurse may often find herself retracing the route she took earlier in the day, especially if she is suddenly given new patients to see.

The district nurse is equivalent in status to a ward sister. An important part of her job is patient assessment. She may be asked to perform a specific function by the medical team, for example dressing an ulcer or removing sutures, but she expects

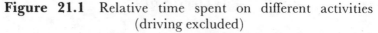

Figure 21.1   Relative time spent on different activities (driving excluded)

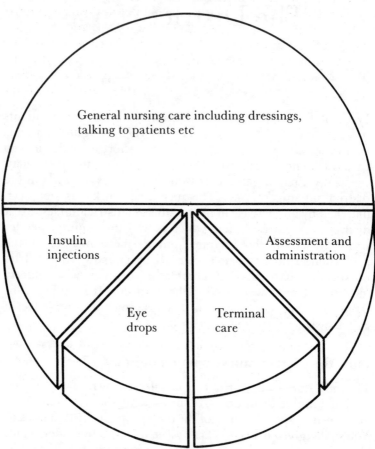

to assess the patient fully physically, socially and psychologically. Sometimes she will call on the home help service, but she may also be supported by her own team. Thus there will be part-time district nurses who do nursing procedures, who are paid as staff nurses, but who do not do initial assessments. The district nurse will also supervise bathing attendants, whose task is to help elderly patients have a weekly bath. Usually, however, she will do much of the work herself. It is the practical nature of the job that is its biggest appeal.

Working with the patient's family

The district nurse's most important resource is the patient's family. They have to do most of the nursing as the district nurse will spend only a very small amount of time in any one home. The relatives can do such tasks as helping the patient in and out of bed, on and off commodes and with washing and mouth care. This means they have to learn how to support the patient physically; only a few of them will be able actually to lift the patient. When a patient is chronically disabled, for example a relatively young person with multiple sclerosis or rheumatoid arthritis, relatives can learn many skills, such as blanket bathing or managing pressure areas, dealing with colostomy bags and even using hoists to lift the patient out of bed. These have to be taught by the district nurse. The district nurse must therefore be a good communicator, and willing to spend time teaching relatives. Furthermore, the relatives will expect her to be able to advise them on such things as diet and bowels, the taking of drugs and how much the patient should do.

Who the district nurse is responsible to

The district nursing service, like the health visitor service, is based on the area health authority, which is responsible for paying the nurses and providing funds for them to run their cars. A district nursing manager supervises the district nursing sisters, district staff nurses and others who are usually part-time.

What the district nurse dislikes doing

Sitting in queues of traffic and doing paper work are the two least liked aspects of the job. The paper work is inevitable and the district nurses often complain that nobody, least of all the doctors, even reads what has been written. Driving about the town can, however, be reduced if other members of the primary health care team make an effort to get messages to the district nurse early enough in the day.

CHAPTER 22

The Practice Manager

There is a difference between management and administration. Management is to do with motivation and change, whereas administration is about keeping things running smoothly and everybody well informed. A practice manager has to be good at both management and administration; he or she must act as a leader in maintaining high standards in the team and must also monitor everything that the team does as unobtrusively as possible. It is said that good administration is invisible, which means that everybody knows where they should be and what they should be doing without feeling they have to make an effort to do so.

Problems arise in management when there have to be changes. The changes will be resisted if people fear that they may be given extra work when they are already overloaded, or that they may lose their job. It is up to the practice manager to identify these fears and explore them properly before trying to make changes. People have also got to understand the reasons for changes; for instance, what are the advantages of installing a computer or making up a disease index?

Other problems that arise in a practice are personality clashes. The practice manager has a key role in sorting out problems between members of the team before they reach crisis level. Good recruiting is important and when a new person is being taken on it is vital that the people he or she is going to work with have a say in his or her selection.

Qualifications

There is still no career structure for practice managers. Many come into primary health care from jobs elsewhere, particularly men who have had a career in the services. There are now problems for people doing this in that there is a basic qualification available for practice managers, the AMSPAR Diploma, which they *may* have to have before they have their pay reimbursed from the family practitioner committee. This development will probably mean that more people will become practice managers after having worked at the reception desk, and although it may lead to a more professional approach there is a risk that there will be a loss of the many useful insights that a career elsewhere can bring.

Pay

The practice manager is paid by the partnership, usually at Whitley Council Executive Officer Grade. The partnership then claims 70% reimbursement from the family practitioner committee. This means that the practice manager is responsible to the partners.

Job Description

Primary objective

The primary objective is to provide administrative support to the partners in respect of staff, premises and finance.

Personal duties

1. *Staff* Some staff will be under the direct supervision of the practice manager, in particular the secretaries and perhaps a filing clerk; but others such as the reception staff who make appointments, look after notes and deal with repeat prescriptions will have their supervision *delegated to the senior receptionist.*
2. *Contracts of employment* have to be prepared for all staff and kept up to date under the terms of the Employment Act of 1978 and subsequent amendments.
3. *Leave* The practice manager will have to check leave entitlement, and keep appropriate records and arrange relief staff where necessary.
4. *Appointing new staff* This is largely the responsibility of the practice manager, who has to draw up application forms

Figure 22.1   Relative time spent on different activites

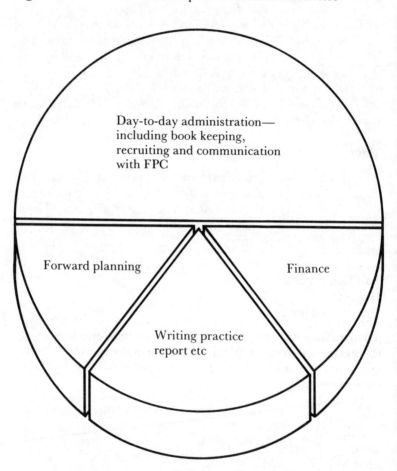

Day-to-day administration—
including book keeping,
recruiting and communication
with FPC

Forward planning

Finance

Writing practice
report etc

and brief job details, advertise posts, make up short lists for
interview, take up references, and arrange interviews. The
usual appointment committee will be the practice manager
and a partner or member of the team who will work with the
new recruit.

5. *Training* The practice manager must ensure that new
   members of staff receive adequate training either by sending
   them on courses or by providing in-service training where
   possible.

Premises

The practice manager is responsible for the premises, which means the fabric of the building, its long term maintenance and its day-to-day maintenance, including making sure it is properly cleaned. The practice manager is responsible for safety and acts as the designated safety officer. This will include checking fire alarm points regularly and holding random fire drills.

Finance

The practice manager has to look after the petty cash, manage the surgery accounts, do the book keeping, sort out PAYE, pay staff salaries and send in claims to the family practitioner committee. These claims have to be made quarterly, or half yearly in the case of rates, and form the major component of the practice financial turnover. This part of the job is likely to occupy a lot of time.

Meetings

The practice manager is expected to be at the monthly partners' meeting and to run and chair a weekly staff meeting. He is expected to minute decisions made at the weekly meeting, but a partner normally keeps the minutes for the partners' monthly meeting.

The use of time by a manager is difficult to estimate as much of the day is quite correctly taken up with many small tasks, usually one or two minute discussions with people. These unplanned meetings are the basic activity of management and what he has been appointed to do.

Complaints

Although a complaints procedure has to be written into all job descriptions most complaints, both from the general public and the staff, will be handled by the practice manager. The usual pattern is to say that, when the practice manager cannot resolve the problem, it is to be taken to a partner who brings it to the next partners' meeting.

Health and Safety Act and public liability
All employers have to make sure that their premises are safe to work in. The responsibility for this usually devolves on the practice manager, whose job includes checking the premises for places where accidents could occur, such as slippery floors. Adequate insurance cover for accidents by staff or the public who may use the building has to be provided and the certificate of insurance displayed.

CHAPTER 23

Social Workers and the Primary Health Care Team

The work of the primary health care team and of the social workers overlaps in several ways. In theory the two teams are complementary to each other; in practice it is surprising how often they will be doing exactly the same things.

Firstly, they tend to deal with the same sections of the population—the vulnerable groups: small children, indeed all children, the elderly and the homeless. They also have special responsibilities for the insane. Secondly, there has been an increase in understanding between the two groups so that social workers and doctors have begun to appreciate each other's limitations and strengths. This has led to a willingness to take on each other's tasks when it is possible to do so effectively. Thirdly, doctors in particular have learnt much from social workers about how to help people help themselves. Probably the biggest intellectual change that has occurred in primary health care is the concept of the Balint group. Balint developed his techniques from his work with groups of social workers when he was teaching about marriage guidance.

There have been and are so many changes in the organisation of the social services that it has become difficult for outsiders to understand how they function. Some of the changes result from a different conception of what a given job involves, but others are due to changes in the law which affect the social services. Much of what they do is regulated by Acts of Parliament. From time to time and in response to public outcry, Parliament will decide that certain groups are particularly at risk. They often respond to this by requiring the social services department to set up registers of such people and to supervise them regularly. This adds to the work of the department, not always with discernible benefits. The problem is made worse because, even where cases of, say child abuse, are discovered, much time and effort has to be expended collecting evidence which is legally watertight. This is because even a Supervision Order can be made only by a Juvenile Court.

Children

The idea that otherwise apparently normal and caring parents could sometimes injure and even murder their children is relatively new. The ignorant, poor and stupid might have hit their children about, but not the well dressed relatively affluent modern parent. Unfortunately being a well heeled adult does not rule out a background of childhood deprivation, either physical or emotional. The scars of such a childhood may result in that person finding it difficult to form relationships with his or her own children which can culminate in him/her actually injuring them.

At the moment society recognises that battering occurs. Fortunately, we have now reached a much greater awareness of sexual abuse in children. This abuse is a damaging problem because the child is put in the position of either colluding with the abuse or reporting it, causing the parent disgrace and probably a prison sentence. The resulting dilemma may be insupportable. Now a third category of child is being recognised, the emotionally deprived child. During the Second World War many children were evacuated out of the big cities because of the risk of bombing; some of these children were later shown to have been emotionally damaged by the experience and later work on children who had spent time in institutions has confirmed this.[1] It has taken over a quarter of a century for emotional deprivation to be accepted by lawyers as something which actually exists. Even nowadays, with widespread knowledge of birth control, including termination of early pregnancy virtually on demand, there are still children born who are not really wanted. They may be wanted by one parent, but not by the other. Mothers who are coerced into having a baby may have great difficulties in the early stages. The situation can then get steadily worse. Such children are given the bare necessities in the way of being fed and clothed but do not have the human contact or encouragement that is needed for normal development.

Case work with children

The social services hear of children at risk from several sources. Where there is a suspicion of battering the child will probably have been admitted to hospital for observation either through the primary health care team or from the Accident and Emergency Department of a hospital. The social worker attached to the hospital paediatric department then hears of the case. Other sources of information are members of the public, perhaps neighbours, or the National Society for the Prevention of Cruelty to Children.

The next phase is for a particular social worker to accept responsibility for the family and to start doing case work. This involves seeing the family involved and starting to piece together the various relationships. This is usually done in the family's home. Asking people about whether they have battered their child might seem like an invitation to be rejected or snubbed. Although parents will sometimes at first deny that there has been anything amiss, they do not always do so and many parents may have realised for a long time that all has not been as they would like in their relationship with the child. These parents may be relieved that they will now be able to talk to somebody outside the family and that positive efforts will be made to do something about it. Parents who batter come from all social classes and include professional people such as solicitors and doctors.

The social worker will be responsible for collecting as much information as possible about the case and it is likely that he or she will then call a case conference which will include the health visitors, general practitioner, hospital staff and, possibly, a representative from the police. A decision then has to be made as to whether there will be a court case or whether the family can be more closely supervised by the social worker and the primary health care team.

The case conference may and usually does nominate someone to be the key worker. This may be the social worker, GP, health visitor or another appropriate professional, who may already be involved with the family.

Care orders and fostering

Once a child is considered at risk the family will need to be counselled and the child seen regularly to make sure that all is well. Children on the 'At Risk Register' are reviewed regularly and are not taken off until all those involved agree there is no further problem. This includes health visitors and doctors. If the situation is more serious and the case has gone to court there are two alternatives. The first is that a Supervision Order will be made requiring the social worker to see and report on the family at regular intervals. This has the advantage that the child stays in his or her own family which will now have the support of the social worker. The other alternative is that the child is taken into care.

Taking a child into care can be a major decision as children sometimes do better even in a deficient family of their own than they do in an institution or even with foster parents. Even the best foster parents can produce young men who drift into a life of petty and not so petty crime and women who become pregnant in their early teens and go on to perpetuate the cycle of deprivation.

This may not be due to fostering; there is very little evidence that it is. For a child in care, adolescence and young adulthood can be particularly difficult times and many of them may need further support beyond the age of 18 when they cease to be legally in care.

Short term fostering

Of all children in care, most come into care for short periods and usually at their parents' request. Sometimes it is because the parents are ill or have to go into hospital, but more often it is because the parents cannot cope and need a temporary break.

The homeless

The housing department has a responsibility to find accommodation for people who have nowhere to live. This was the responsibility of the social services until the Homeless Persons Act. All the same, social workers with their many vulnerable clients are still often involved as well.

Nowadays most of the homeless are single people, many of whom would, not long ago, have been settled down in a mental hospital as long-stay patients. Others are part of a floating population that seems unable to cope with normal life even when times are good and employment high.

Homeless people tend to congregate in the big cities. They usually have multiple health problems, including infestations and tuberculosis. They have difficulty in getting treatment because as they have no fixed address doctors treat them as temporary residents and in many cases fail to give them continuity of care. Many such people live in squats but others are provided with accommodation either in hostels or in night shelters. Despite considerable efforts to provide occupation, as against employment, many of them seem unable to do more than drift through each day.

There are many fewer drifting homeless women than men, but there are increasing numbers of women who leave their husbands because of violence. The violence may not have been increasing; the women may just have become aware that help is available. Battered wives are usually placed in refuges, sometimes many miles from where they normally live and almost always in inconspicuous buildings. The aim is to make it impossible for their husbands to come to molest them. Refuges are intended only for short stays of up to six months until the quarrel is resolved or proper housing can be found. Sometimes several families with young children stay in one home together and this can lead to outbreaks of diarrhoea and other health hazards. Such homes need a lot of support and help from the primary health care team.

The elderly

Between 65 and 75 years most people can manage easily in their own homes without any support except from their own families. After 75, however, increasing numbers find it impossible to cope, not necessarily because of any specific illness but because of increasing physical and mental weakness. A crisis then tips the balance.

Where they cannot manage in their own homes they may manage in accommodation specifically designed for the elderly, normally with a residential warden. This may be privately owned or provided by the council. The social worker's role here may be no more than to negotiate and organise the move. Once again the social worker will have first looked for other solutions such as home helps, day care, volunteer support and so on.

Part three accommodation

The name 'part three' originates from the section of the National Assistance Act 1948 that decreed that such accommodation should be provided. Part three are residential homes housing people who, although not incontinent, are in need of some care. The original idea was that part three was explicitly not for people needing nursing care. This is now changing and part three homes are taking some who are more disabled and dependent.

Part three homes do become their residents' 'home'. If residents fall ill and have to go into hospital their room in the part three home is kept open for them. As well as providing food and shelter the care staff at the home will also try to make sure that there are entertainments, outings and support. If a person is too ill to be looked after in part three accommodation he or she has to be admitted to a long-term hospital bed. Such cases are rare because of the expense of hospitals and because part three is more humane.

Some part three accommodation is set aside for short stays. This is to give temporary relief to people who live in the community and more especially to those who look after them. This concept of respite care, and also of day care in part three homes, is all part of the policy of trying to keep people living in the community as long as possible.

The physically and mentally handicapped

Although the number of severely physically handicapped children has decreased over the last two decades it seems that a higher proportion survive into adolescence. There are fewer with cerebral palsy, perhaps as a result of better obstetric care, but more who have paraplegia due to spina bifida. There are more severely disabled survivors from road traffic accidents and from strokes. These young people may live at home and come in daily to workshops, but many of them are too badly affected for their relatives to cope. The answer is to set up hostels for the disabled, often adjacent to the workshops. Such hostels will have resident wardens and be well enough staffed to cope with severely disabled people. Once again the objective is to make the hostel the patients' home and to provide them with separate bedrooms or even flatlets that they can manage themselves. The hostels are set up and run by the social services departments.

Mentally handicapped people have for many years been looked after in large hospitals, often in the middle of the countryside, usually in old listed country houses. The present policy is to close such hospitals and move the people in them back into the community, perhaps into houses in the centre of towns where they can do more to look after themselves, do their own shopping and become independent. Setting up such households and their supervision has become the responsibility of the social services.

The social worker and the Mental Health Act 1983

The Mental Health Act of 1983 deals with people who need to be admitted to mental hospitals. Under Sections 2, 3 and 4, approved social workers have to be consulted and certify that admission is necessary, but under the terms of the Act the social worker has the statutory obligation to look for alternative ways of dealing with the problem. It is not his or her job to question the diagnosis or proposed treatment but to discuss with the nearest relative whether there is some alternative to the person being admitted to a mental hospital. The nearest relative is precisely defined in the Act.

If the admission is under Section 2 the nearest relative has no right of veto over the social worker's application. If the application is under Section 3, for treatment, the nearest relative can override the social worker, who must then apply to the county court if he still wishes to admit the patient.

The home care service—home helps

The home care service is often referred to as the 'home help service'. The change in name is a result of change in emphasis, from looking after the home to looking after the person.

The home care service is organised by the social services. The usual pattern is for there to be an area home care organiser who runs the service and who has to be contacted if it is felt that a patient needs a home help. There is then an assessment visit to decide how frequently home help is needed and the tasks to be done. Any patient who has a home help may have to make a contribution towards the cost, according to his or her means; this obviously does not apply if he or she is on Supplementary Benefit.

Home care workers do housework and shopping, go to the chemist and perform other simple tasks. Although they are not nurses and do not do nursing tasks, the borderline is vague and they do sometimes do what could be called auxiliary nursing.

In some areas an extended service is provided so that for a short time the home care service will replace a relative—for example, if the more able bodied of an elderly couple has to go into hospital. This may involve going in two or three times a day, supervising tablets, helping people to bed and so on.

Reference

1 Bowlby, J. (1953) *Child care and the growth of love*. London, Pelican.

CHAPTER 24

Care of the Dying

The extended team

Managing dying patients involves a more extended group than the conventional primary health care team. If death is managed properly, vital roles are those of the relatives, especially the husband or wife, and the other professional but non-medical people such as clergymen and lawyers. All these people have to be dealt with honestly if they are to be effective and it is possible to do this only if there is honesty with the patient. This is a good reason for making sure that the patient knows that he or she is seriously ill and dying. If the patient does not know this, many members of the team cannot be brought in. It is up to the doctor to get over this hurdle and, for what it is worth, it seems that by the time most people are told they are dying they have already guessed it and are glad to have it out in the open.

The aims of the team

1. The first aim is to keep the patient functioning as normally as possible, for as long as possible. He or she may have things he wishes to do while he still has time, for example tidying up his affairs or going somewhere he has not so far had the opportunity to visit, but had always meant to see.
2. This aim will gradually be overtaken by the next, which is to keep the person comfortable. Not just free of pain, but also not sick or constipated. Eventually he or she will be confined to bed but until then shortness of breath, incontinence and weakness all need to be alleviated.
3. The last aim is coming to terms with the sadness of dying. The dying person needs time to come to terms with actually dying and his or her spouse needs time to get used to his or her going. There is also the fear of death.

The problems of isolation, anxiety and fear used to be ignored in conventional medical training and the legacy of this is that many people still feel considerable resentment at the way general practitioners have handled the care of their dying relatives.[1]

Activities of daily living

Dying people cannot cope because of:

1. *Pain* Remember that they often have more than one pain. Adequate pain relief must be constant.
2. *Nausea and vomiting* Again, it is usually possible to control these symptoms. Sometimes their underlying cause can be found, but it is more important to get on and relieve the symptoms than to fuss about whether it is due to raised calcium or urea concentrations or whatever.
3. *Constipation* Although manipulating laxatives usually achieves normal bowel action, sometimes the patient needs the district nurse to help with enemas or a gentle manual removal. Communication between the doctor and the district nurse is essential here, as the aim is to avoid such a drastic remedy if possible.
4. *Incontinence* Fortunately there are now disposable catheters and bags available that make it possible for men to carry on for years with an indwelling catheter. The position is not so good for women, but for both sexes it may be possible to cope by using incontinence pads, especially in the last few days of life.
5. *Weakness* Although this may be due to the disease or drugs, it can also be due to inactivity and boredom. A physiotherapist can often help, or an occupational therapist.

(It is not my intention to write about the detailed management of the dying patient as this book is more about the problems of team work. The subject has been dealt with brilliantly elsewhere.[2] Stott and Finlay's *Care of the Dying* cannot be recommended too highly.)

Communication between team members

The problem when somebody is dying is that most of the team will be involved as the situation develops stage by stage, but there may never be a time when a formal meeting such as a case conference is appropriate. The doctor is the person who has to decide such things as to whether the patient needs to go into hospital or which drugs are to be prescribed. He or she has therefore got to make sure that he or she is *accessible* either by telephone or in person. Many doctors who run out-of-hours rotas make an exception for dying patients. Most doctors will accept telephone calls from nurses and hospice workers at any reasonable time of the day or in the evening at home.

If the doctor and district nurse, or hospice nurse, can meet at the patient's bedside this will help the family feel that they are being looked after by a team rather than by a succession of individuals.

Who can be involved at which stages

Although the length of time may be different for different cancers or other lethal diseases, patients nevertheless move through a series of stages. At first they are fully mobile if symptoms such as severe pain or breathlessness can be controlled, and they will lead an almost normal life. In due course weakness or some other incapacitating symptom will keep them to their house. The next phase is being bedbound, and once this point has been reached they will often rapidly go into a final phase, when they will lapse into unconsciousness and die.

Early phase after diagnosis

Inevitably it will be the doctor who is involved when the diagnosis is made and it is up to him to start contacting other team members. Where there has been surgery involving the removal of, say, a breast or bowel, specialist nurses may have already been advising about a prosthesis or appliances. It is the doctor, however, who has to make contact with the spouse and start offering the services of the other members of the team. Once it is realised that death is going to come soon, people go through a series of well recognised reactions. Often they start feeling angry and resentful and looking for reasons why it should happen to them. The next phase is one of bargaining with fate; this changes into acceptance and depression and then perhaps acceptance with tranquility. Both partners go through these stages and may wish to share them. Where death is sudden the survivor will have to go through the stages of grieving on his or her own, which may be more difficult and often includes resentment of the partner who is not there to share it.

Although it may not seem right to introduce a hospice worker to the family before they have fully accepted the disease, the benefits often outweigh the disadvantages. Long experience and training enable hospice workers to handle the powerful emotions present and they can sometimes help people to recognise what their own feelings actually are. These can then be worked through.

Many people fear not so much the fact that they are going to die, but how they will die. They have visions of suffocation or of great agony and struggle. A visit by the hospice nurse gives them an opportunity to discuss this and also, if they are single people, for them to be offered support at the actual moment of death. When a patient dies in a hospice great efforts are made to ensure that somebody is with him or her until he or she goes.

Being housebound

No rigid lines are drawn between being in a hospice and being at home. Where possible most people would rather die at home and this is the present trend. Sometimes, however, the patient's relatives need a break, or his or her drug regimen needs modification so as to make sure there is adequate relief of pain. It is then appropriate for him or her to go into a hospice for a short spell.

The district nurse can give much help and support as soon as the patient reaches the stage of being unable to get out. They can advise on pressure areas and arrange for bathing and for such things as urinals and commodes. Where a domiciliary physiotherapist is available, he or she can sometimes offer advice, but an occupational therapist has been trained to help over a much wider range of activities of daily living.

Even if there is a willing relative able to help the patient dress or bathe, the patient may wish to retain his or her independence for as long as possible. An occupational therapist can sometimes help a woman go on cooking occasional meals, and to look after herself and do various other things that she has always done. This will help her keep her stake in society for that little bit longer.

Bedbound

Being bedbound is the next phase and it is to be deferred as long as possible because the support required for somebody who spends a day in bed is so very much greater. Only if the dying person's spouse is able, strong and has no other commitments, can this stage go on for very long; even the most willing relatives can become totally exhausted. This will add guilt to the already heavy emotional burden being carried by the dying person.

Meals on wheels, laundry services, loans of equipment and so on can alleviate the situation, but unless the dying person's relatives can be given an occasional holiday they will end up with an unnecessary hospital death. Although most hospital consultants are willing to admit the dying to hospital for a short time to give the relatives a rest, a hospice nurse who can co-ordinate admission into a hospice and also visit the patient at home is in a better position to judge the right moment for doing things.

Terminal phase

As the patient lapses into coma so the normal team of district nurses and relatives becomes less able to cope. In these circumstances a Marie Curie nurse may be asked to sit with the patient at night. These nurses are paid from the funds of the Marie Curie Foundation and the district nurse is empowered to ask them to start coming. As they are paid out of a limited budget they usually cannot spend more than one or two nights with the patient. This is a disadvantage as it is often difficult to say exactly when a patient is going to die, and by the time the Marie Curie nurse is called in and arrives, the patient is sometimes only minutes from death.

The clergy and religious aspects of dying

It is unusual for Church of England clergy to be present at the time of death; indeed any expression of religiosity at the time of death seems to be regarded among the British as in slightly bad taste. Hindus, however, will expect their Holy Book (Bhagvad Gita) to be read to them when they are dying. Muslims should face Mecca and should have prayers whispered to them by their relatives. It is important that team members know about and understand that different cultures have different ways of coping with death. It is also necessary that they try to give relatives an honest assessment of how much longer they expect the dying person to live as arrangements have to be made for last rites, and in the case of Muslims the body must be buried within 24 hours.

From time to time team members will be asked to act as witnesses to Wills. It need hardly be said that when this happens they are being asked to exercise their professional judgement that the person signing the Will is of sound mind and knows what he or she is doing. This is particularly important for Wills made at the end of life because if they are disputed it can easily be argued that the Will was signed under some sort of duress.

A special relationship with the dying

People die at all hours of the day and night and it is not possible for any team member to undertake to be available to give support throughout the whole 24 hours. Sometimes a close relationship with a particular member of the team is formed and this can lead to considerable stress and feelings of guilt when the team member feels unable to cope, especially if he or she feels that he is expected to attend during the night as death approaches.

One way round this is to try to forewarn relatives if death is coming. There is no absolute need for a doctor to come and certify death as soon as it has occurred: the relatives can usually tell if someone has died. Their concern is whether the doctor or nurse who knows the patient will be available if something unexpected occurs. One way round the difficulty is for the medical attendant to offer a visit late in the evening, even if he or she is not actually the duty doctor or nurse. Sometimes an injection of morphine given by the last visitor will help to settle the patient for the night. This contact with the relatives who are looking after the patient during the night often gives them that bit of support that they need, and from the doctor's point of view these planned late evening visits are not arduous and are often very rewarding.

References

1 Wilkes, E. (1984) Dying now *Lancet* **i**; 950–2.
2 Stott, N.C.H. and Finlay, I.G. (1984) *Care of the dying*. Edinburgh, Churchill Livingstone.

CHAPTER 25

Protocols

This section consists of protocols for the management of different conditions in general practice. They are set out as used and are therefore written in such a way that any member of the team can understand what we are trying to do and how.

These protocols are not meant to be the last word on the subject, but merely to act as baselines for any primary care team to start building up their own library. Medical care and management are effective only if they are frequently reviewed and often changed.

The term protocol may need some explanation. Broadly it means a statement of how a primary health care team intends to deal with a particular disease. The use of the word is relatively new and probably derives from the Oxford English Dictionary definition *"a formal or official statement of a transaction or proceeding"*.

The advantage of a protocol is that it means that members of the team such as the practice nurse know what the overall pattern of management is going to be and how they should manage at each stage. A subsidiary advantage of setting up a protocol is that the discussion involved teaches everybody something about the disease and enables them to formulate a more logical pattern of management.

The disadvantage of a protocol is that it may lead to excessive rigidity, this is why it has to be set out partly in the form of a discussion. It is not intended that all patients should be treated in exactly the same way, but rather that there should be guidelines on their management.

Protocols are used for scientific experiments, but they then have to be adhered to rigidly, especially over such issues as which patients are to be reunited, how they are to be randomised and so on. This is because if mistakes are made the scientific value of the exercise is compromised. Such constraints do not apply when the aim is to improve the treatment and comfort of a population in the care of the team.

In Chapter 3 I pointed out that in managing chronic disease it was helpful to:

1. Set out the objectives.
2. Decide whether it was worthwhile having a separate clinic for a particular condition.
3. Devise a flow chart that would enable the objectives to be achieved.
4. Create a morbidity index for procedural review.
5. Devise decision charts or a clinical algorithm if there are management decisions to be made.

We felt it was only worthwhile having a clinic for diabetic patients. Other chronic illnesses were best fitted in with normal length appointments with the practice nurse. Diabetic patients take longer and the doctor has also got to be available.

The flow chart is important. A number of drug houses supply free charts. It is worthwhile trying out a flow chart before finally adopting it.

MANAGEMENT OF HYPERTENSION

Introduction

Blood pressure varies from person to person and also gets higher with age. In one sense therefore there is no such thing as a normal blood pressure; all that can be said is that as it gets higher so people are more likely to get strokes and heart attacks. Treatment prevents strokes but has less influence on death rates from heart disease. Treatment also has side effects; some of these are from the drugs, but others are from the fact that the patient begins to feel he is unwell because he knows he has raised blood pressure.

There is no way of knowing you have high blood pressure except by getting somebody to take it for you. It it a myth that high blood pressure causes headaches. Not merely does blood presure not give you headaches, but it may even make some people feel extremely well. This means that as a team we have two problems. Firstly we have to identify those with higher than

Figure 25.1   Algorithm for the management of hypertension

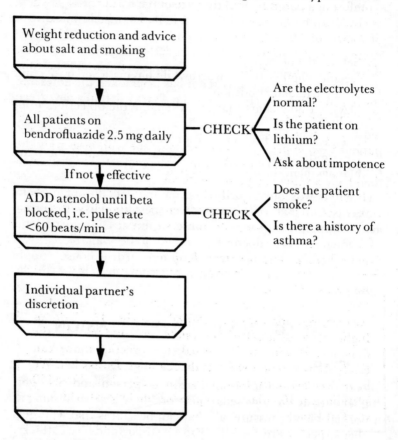

average blood pressure and, secondly, we have to decide which ones we are going to treat.

Identifying patients with high blood pressure

As most people see their doctor about twice a year it should be possible to find out which of them have high blood pressure, just by making sure that their blood pressure is taken when they come for an appointment. In most cases it will be normal and then all that needs to be done is to put a marker in the notes to remind the doctor to take it again in five years' time. There is no point in checking it sooner as it rarely goes up that quickly.

We have started by 'flagging' the notes of all patients whom we want to check – that is, all men and women between the ages of 25 and 65, though we may extend this list. The 'flag' is a red piece of cardboard which sticks out of the top of the notes. This draws the attention of the doctor or nurse to the need to take the patient's blood pressure. When it has been taken the notes and the flag are left in the clerical assistant's tray so that a new green flag can be inserted, inscribed with a date five years on indicating when the next blood pressure check is due. If the patient's blood pressure is raised he or she will be seen by the practice nurse, who will take over management. The notes will then have a yellow flag put into them.

In due course the majority of our patients will have a green or yellow flag and we will be able to write to those with red flags to invite them to come for a blood pressure check.

Treating those with a yellow flag

Note for reception staff
You will have seen that the blood pressure is recorded as two figures, for example 120/80 mm Hg. The 120, or higher reading, is called the systolic level and the 80 is the diastolic. If you are interested, the practice nurse can easily show you how she gets the readings. Do ask her. We have decided for the time being that the levels of above 150 systolic and 105 diastolic represent the level at which to start treatment.

As many people's blood pressure goes up if they are anxious it is worth while taking it three times on separate days before doing anything else. This may result in a normal reading, in which case the patient can be green-flagged to be seen in one year. Sometimes the blood pressure is high because the patient is overweight. Dieting can reduce the weight and also the blood pressure. Again, if this is effective the patient can be green-flagged for one year.

This will leave a final group of patients who will be under the practice nurse's care for regular checks on their blood pressure and tablets. Before treatment is started, and every year thereafter, they will have their urine checked and a blood sample taken for blood urea and electrolyte analysis. The follow-up of blood urea and electrolytes is most conveniently done in the month of their birthday. This spreads the workload for the practice round the year and acts as a convenient reminder of when it should be done. We used to do an ECG on all patients but found this was never a help in the management so we have now stopped doing it. The doctor will also need to examine the patient properly before treatment begins. A normal length 10 minute appointment is enough.

The doctors

The check list is intended as a reminder. It is up to the doctors to modify it according to changes in medical thinking. For the first six months of the new set up an ECG was taken of every patient but the practice nurse pointed out that the doctor tended to look at it briefly and in any case no decisions to treat or not to treat, or indeed to do anything else, were made on the basis of the tracing. It may be that there are other aspects of the long term management of people with hypertension that need to be amended in the same way.

Usually all patients are cared for by their own doctor. The exception is when there is a trainee in the practice who may identify a hypertensive patient and wish to start treating him. It is helpful if the trainee has guidelines on what drugs to start with and this is one place where a practice policy would be useful. When partners cannot agree to commit themselves to using a particular regimen they can sometimes agree on what would be an appropriate starting regimen for the trainee to use.

The practice nurse and treating blood pressure

Much of the work of treating hypertension devolves onto the practice nurse, who not only has to do a series of routine tests at the beginning of treatment but also has to continue long term supervision. After trying several designs of cards for record keeping, including graphics and elaborate layouts for taking the history, we eventually settled for a simple pale blue card with vertically ruled columns for date, weight, blood pressure and comments.

Patients need only to be seen twice a year once the dose of treatment needed to control their blood pressure has been found. Ask them to come in their birthday month and again about six months later, i.e. if born in January, come in January and July.

If at review session the blood pressure has altered, their treatment should not be altered immediately, instead they should have further blood pressure readings taken over the next few weeks and then if it is persistently different the drugs can be modified.

If in doubt, for instance if the blood pressure has suddenly soared, the nurse should let the patient's own doctor know.

Adding further drugs

The traditional approach to the management of blood pressure was to increase the dose until the blood pressure was controlled or the patient suffered side effects. If the blood pressure was still poorly controlled another drug would be added on. Another aspect is to think of substituting an alternative. Calcium channel blocking agents and angiotensin inhibitors are more effective in some patients.

These two different styles have been described as 'stepwise' treatment and 'tailor made'.

THYROID DISEASE

Identifying patients at risk

A register is kept of all patients on thyroid tablets. A second register is kept of all patients who have been treated for an overactive thryoid (hyperthyroidism). Both groups should be reviewed annually. A check list is made up each month to enable this to be done.

Repeat prescriptions

When a patient is on thyroid tablets it is easier to check if he or she has been reviewed because he or she will probably be having regular repeat prescriptions. When the prescription is issued the notes should be checked to see when the patient last had his or her blood tested. These systems are all now built in to the repeat prescribing package in the computer.

Note for receptionists

The thyroid gland is situated in the neck and it controls the rate at which the body functions. If the thyroid hormone which is secreted by the gland becomes deficient the patient will slow down, gain weight and eventually die. It can also overact, when the patient becomes over-active and again may die. Fortunately it is now possible to measure the exact level of thyroid hormone in the blood, which helps diagnosis and can be used to monitor treat-ment. The majority of the patients in the practice who have thyroid disease have a lack of thyroid hormone and therefore now have to have it in tablet form. The blood level needs to be checked annually to make sure the dose is correct and the patient is taking the tablets correctly. This is to be done in their birthday month. When the thyroid gland has been overactive and the patient has had treat-ment with radioactive iodine it can then lapse into under-activity. It is thought that every year one in 10 such patients who have been treated for an overactive thyroid become underactive. The task of the team is to look for these patients, especially as the condition is so slow in the onset that many may never realise what is happening even when they have been warned about it.

DIABETES

What are we trying to achieve?

There is increasing evidence that poor control of diabetes results in more complications. Diabetes is still the commonest cause of blindness in this country among those under 60 and this blindness is now largely preventable. Some diabetics manage their disease well and know a lot about it but others try to ignore the condition and neglect themselves. It is this second group that needs the help of the primary health care team and they are the people who get lost in yet another collusion of anonymity.

Our aims are therefore:

1. To try to make sure that we have identified all the diabetics in the practice and that they are seen at least twice each year.
2. To make sure all diabetics know about the importance of having their eyes checked regularly for early retinopathy, the risks of poor control, the dangers of injury if they have neuropathy and the bad effects of smoking.
3. To try to monitor blood sugar concentrations consistently and maintain them below 10 ml/l and maintain a glycosylated haemoglobin level of below 10%.

Table 25.1 Expected number of diabetics in a practice of 7500

Age (years)	Expected	No. in practice
Under 20	15	
20–29	9	
30–39	15	
40–49	15	
50–59	12	
60 and over	9	

Definition of diabetes according to the World Health Organization is a random blood sugar concentration of over 11 ml/l. We would usually be taking a specimen of blood about one hour after a meal.

Registration and identification of patients

The register will be maintained by the practice manager who will also monitor attendance at the clinics. Patients will be identified:

1. As they are diagnosed.
2. When they register as new patients from other practices.
3. From the repeat prescribing list when they ask for insulin or oral hypoglycaemics.

About half the diabetics in the population are undiagnosed and at the present we are not doing a screening clinic except

Figure 25.2 Diabetic surveillance

Date	Smokes?	Seen optician Yes/No	Inspect Syringes	Feet	Weight	B.P.	Bl. Sugar Series	Acuity/ Fundoscopy	Medication a.m. p.m.
	N	N	N	N	N	N	N	D	D
	Always	Annually	6 mthly	6 mthly	6 mthly	Annually	Annually	Annually	Annually

Explanation
N = Nurse
D = Doctor

when we ask obese patients attending the practice nurse to bring a specimen of urine to test for sugar.

Holding a clinic

Patients will be identified from the register by the practice manager and names checked with the doctor they are registered with. To help spread the clinics through the year they will be asked to come for the first time in their birthday month, or six months from their birthday month. Thus a patient born in January will be invited in January and July.

Patients' notes

As diabetic patients' notes tend to get rather bulky a separate folder is kept of information directly pertaining to their diabetes. A blue cardboard sticker in a patient's notes reminds the receptionist that that patient is diabetic and the notes can then be made available every time a patient makes an ordinary appointment to see the doctor.

The flow chart in the patient's diabetic folder is to remind the nurse and doctor at the clinic what they should be looking for and checking at each attendance.

Additional checklist

Some things are kept on the flow chart (Figure 25.2) on the principle that they need continuous reinforcement. This applies above all to cigarette smoking, which has a much greater effect on the circulation of diabetics than on other people. It does not just add on to the effects of the arteries of diabetics but seems to multiply the effect. There are other things that are worth remembering, such as asking patients if they have joined the Diabetic Association.

Syringe checks

It is worth looking at the syringes of diabetics to make sure that these are not wearing out and also to make sure that their users are drawing up insulin to the level specified in the notes. This is less of a problem than it used to be now that all insulins are in U100 strengths. A syringe is worn out when the plunger gets too loose for it to support the weight of the barrel if the syringe is held up by its handle.

MANAGEMENT OF EPILEPSY

According to the *British National Formulary*, phenytoin is the recommended drug of choice; carbamazepine can then be added. The problem with these drugs is that they have a narrow therapeutic index. It is essential that the dose is monitored by measuring the blood level until the patient is well controlled. Once the epilepsy is satisfactorily controlled the frequency of doing blood level checks can be left to individual doctors, who would normally see the patient every six months. When a patient is on long term phenytoin there may be a case for checking folic acid levels, but this would be left to the individual's own doctor.

Patients who get side effects or who are poorly controlled on phenytoin and carbamazepine can be tried on sodium valproate. There is no point in monitoring blood levels with sodium valproate as the level in the blood does not equate with the efficiency of the drug.

It is probably better to keep off phenobarbitone as it is now a controlled drug. Benzoadiazepines are usually too sedating and tolerance appears rapidly.

Instructions for receptionists if a patient has an epileptic fit
The longer the patient goes on fitting the more difficult it is to get him or her out of it. If you get a call saying an epileptic is having a fit let his or her doctor know immediately.

Controlling a fit
An injection of diazepam is the quickest way to control a fit. Make sure some 10 mg ampules are available.

Where there is no doctor to give the injection into a vein the patient should be given the diazepam rectally. Patients' relatives could do this or a nurse if the patient is fitting in the surgery and no doctor is about.

Stesolid rectal tubes contain diazepam in rectal solution. This should be in the drug cupboard.

Figure 25.3 Epileptic protocol

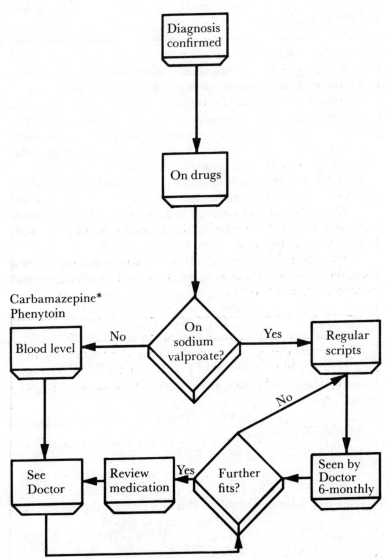

*When the patient is on Carbamazepine or Phenytoin the blood level is important as often there is poor control because the amount in the blood stream is too low. There are also problems with side effects if the level gets too high. Measuring blood levels for sodium valproate is not helpful as the level in the blood seems to bear no relationship to the side effects experienced and the efficacy of the drug.

LONG-TERM MANAGEMENT OF DEPRESSION

Patients on Lithium

Note to receptionist

A few people in the population are subject to what is known as a manic depression psychosis. They are sometimes deeply depressed and almost unable to do anything; at other times they are quite extraordinarily active, sleep little and rush about in an excitable state. The changes in mood occur over a period of weeks but may last for months. Some of these people benefit from taking lithium, which damps down and smooths off the mood swings. It is not known how lithium works.

The problem with lithium is that it has to be given in exactly the right dose. Too much will make the patient feel ill and may endanger his or her life. As different people need different amounts of lithium to keep them stable the only way to check that a patient is getting the correct dose is to do regular tests to check the level in the blood. The correct dose is not constant because different amounts are absorbed by the patient at different times.

Protocol for the management of patients on lithium

The following drugs are lithium salts and are used for treating manic depressive patients:

Camcolit, Liskonum, Phasal, Priadel—all lithium carbonate
Litrarex—lithium citrate

Note they are not interchangeable as they are absorbed at different rates.

If patients are taking these they will need regular blood tests, weekly or more often at first, then every four weeks once the treatment has settled down.

Results of the tests, showing lithium level in the blood, should be put on the repeat prescription card so that the doctor making out the repeat prescription can confirm that it has been done before issuing too many repeat scripts. Usually the medical secretary will look out for the biochemistry results as they arrive in the post and inform the patient by telephone if they are normal. The level aimed for is between 0.6 and 1.2 mmol/l.

Further reading

Waine, C. (1986) Why not care for your diabetic patients? In the Royal College of General Practitioners Diabetic Folder.
Martin, E (1987) Epilepsy—a general practice problem. In the Royal College of General Practitioners Epilepsy folder.

INDEX